Fibromyalgia:

The Complete Guide from Medical Experts and Patients

— •◆• —

Sharon Ostalecki, PhD

JONES AND BARTLETT PUBLISHERS
Sudbury, Massachusetts
BOSTON   TORONTO   LONDON   SINGAPORE

World Headquarters

Jones and Bartlett Publishers	Jones and Bartlett Publishers	Jones and Bartlett Publishers
40 Tall Pine Drive	Canada	International
Sudbury, MA 01776	6339 Ormindale Way	Barb House, Barb Mews
978-443-5000	Mississauga, Ontario L5V 1J2	London W6 7PA
info@jbpub.com	Canada	United Kingdom
www.jbpub.com		

Jones and Bartlett's books and products are available through most bookstores and online booksellers. To contact Jones and Bartlett Publishers directly, call 800-832-0034, fax 978-443-8000, or visit our website www.jbpub.com.

Substantial discounts on bulk quantities of Jones and Bartlett's publications are available to corporations, professional associations, and other qualified organizations. For details and specific discount information, contact the special sales department at Jones and Bartlett via the above contact information or send an email to specialsales@jbpub.com.

The authors, editor, and publisher have made every effort to provide accurate information. However, they are not responsible for errors, omissions, or for any outcomes related to the use of the contents of this book and take no responsibility for the use of the products and procedures described. Treatments and side effects described in this book may not be applicable to all people; likewise, some people may require a dose or experience a side effect that is not described herein. Drugs and medical devices are discussed that may have limited availability controlled by the Food and Drug Administration (FDA) for use only in a research study or clinical trial. Research, clinical practice, and government regulations often change the accepted standard in this field. When consideration is being given to use of any drug in the clinical setting, the health care provider or reader is responsible for determining FDA status of the drug, reading the package insert, and reviewing prescribing information for the most up-to-date recommendations on dose, precautions, and contraindications, and determining the appropriate usage for the product. This is especially important in the case of drugs that are new or seldom used.

Library of Congress Cataloging-in-Publication Data
Fibromyalgia : the complete guide from medical experts and patients / Sharon Ostalecki, editor.
    p. cm.
Includes bibliographical references.
ISBN-13: 978-0-7637-4640-7 (pbk.)
ISBN-10: 0-7637-4640-1 (pbk.)
1. Fibromyalgia--Popular works. I. Ostalecki, Sharon.
RC927.3.O88 2007
616.7'42--dc22
                            2007001168

6048

Production Credits

Executive Publisher: Christopher Davis	Manufacturing Buyer: Therese Connell
Associate Editor: Kathy Richardson	Composition: Arlene Apone
Production Director: Amy Rose	Cover Design: Kristin Ohlin
Production Editor: Tracey Chapman	Cover Image: © John Romans
Senior Marketing Manager: Katrina Gosek	Printing and Binding: Malloy, Inc.
Associate Marketing Manager: Rebecca Wasley	Cover Printing: Malloy, Inc.

Printed in the United States of America
11 10 09   10 9 8 7 6 5 4 3

Dedicated to:

Matthew Philip, Abigail, Isabella, and Jacob

Acknowledgments

"Never, never, never, never give up."
—Winston Churchill

No one manages fibromyalgia without help, let alone manages to write a book to help others who have this confusing disease, and I am no exception.

My thanks must begin with Dr. Martin Tamler, a devoted specialist in the treatment and teaching of fibromyalgia. Back when I was first coming to terms with what having fibromyalgia meant in my life, Dr. Tamler's guidance, patience, and encouragement were invaluable to me. Every patient with a chronic disease begins to run out of hope at one time or another. Dr. Tamler insisted that hope was essential to my progress, and infused me with more whenever my stock ran low. Later on, when I developed a passion for reaching out to other fibromyalgia patients, wanting to share what I had learned, he became my mentor. When Dr. Tamler offered me the opportunity to share the podium with him speaking on fibromyalgia, I knew that an important mission in my life was to educate and help others live with fibromyalgia. It was Dr. Tamler's commitment and dedication that inspired me to undertake this book.

A special thanks to Dr. Peter Ianni for his understanding, and for his support of this book. A special thanks also to Loren DeVinney, my physical therapist for many years, who has an amazing way to tame the "gunk" in a fibromyalgia patient's muscles.

My gratitude goes out to all the professionals whose contributions have made this book possible.

My heartfelt thanks to the many dozens of fibromyalgia patients whom I have met at lectures, and in my practice. Because they shared with me their concerns, pain, and successes, they are largely responsible for my moving forward with this book.

A very special thanks to the contributing patient authors for opening yourselves to me, and telling me about your experience with fibromyalgia including details that were not only personal but sometimes painful.

I appreciate the enthusiastic support of Jones and Bartlett, my publisher, and particularly of Chris Davis, who recognized the importance of a book that identifies the many facets of this perplexing disorder and the importance of a multi-disciplinary approach to the treatment of fibromyalgia.

My editor, Kathy Krajco, sharpened the focus and organization of my thoughts, and redirected me many times. She taught me "many things" beyond the scope of this book. I am very grateful for her guidance throughout.

John Romans took my ideas and turned them into a cover that captures the real meaning of living with FM.

Priscilla Gish is more than a dear friend. She is an adviser and supporter par excellence. For all of it, my thanks.

Finally, the ongoing love and loyalty of my family have meant the world to me. This book belongs to you as much as to me.

Contents

Preface xiii

Contributors xix

Editor's Biography xxiii

CHAPTER 1   Fibromyalgia 1
             Joseph Meerschaert, MD and Peter Ianni, PhD

             Understanding Fibromyalgia 1
             Diagnosis 3
             The Examination 4
             The Causes of Pain in FM 8
             The Treatment Team 9
             A Final Word 14

CHAPTER 2   Fibrolyalgia: A Patient's Perspective 17
             Jane Charlton

CHAPTER 3   Sleep: An Overview 25
             M. Safwan Badr, MD and Anan Salloum, MD

             The Physiology of Sleep 25
             Sleep Disorders 30
             Conclusion 38

CHAPTER 4   Interventional Treatments for Fibromyalgia
             and Other Pain Conditions 41
             Dennis W. Dobritt, DO

             Trigger Point Injections 43
             Nerve Blocks 44
             Spinal Injections 47
             Cryolesioning and Radiofrequency Lesioning 49
             Intervertebral Disc Procedures 50
             Advanced Interventional Therapies 51

CHAPTER 5   Pharmacology Management in Fibromyalgia . . 55
             Randy Schad, RPh

             Drug Therapy 56
             Potential Herbal and Prescription
                 Medication Interaction 70
             Conclusion 70

CHAPTER 6   Growing Up, Living With, and
             Managing Fibromyalgia 73
             Jerry Sauve

CHAPTER 7   Endocrine Dysfunction Concurrent
             with Fibromyalgia 83
             Sander J. Paul, MD

             Thyroid Disease 83
             Adrenal Disease 94
             Conclusions 99

CHAPTER 8   Temporomandibular Disorders (TMD)
             and Facial Pain 103
             Ghabi Kaspo, DDS

             Musculoskeletal Disorders 104
             TMJ Anatomy 105
             Symptoms of TMD 108
             Additional Symptoms Associated with TMD 110
             TMD Treatment 112
             Self-Management 116
             Finding a Specialist 117

CHAPTER **9**   **Irritable Bowel Syndrome (IBS)**
Concurrent with Fibromyalgia 119
Olafur S. Palsson, PsyD and Donald Moss, PhD

The Nature of IBS 120
Demographics 120
Causes of IBS 120
The Impact of IBS 122
IBS and Fibromyalgia 123
Treatment of IBS 125
The Future Direction of Treatment 127

CHAPTER **10**   **Acupuncture in the Management**
of Fibromyalgia 131
Mitchell Elkiss, DO

The Ancient Theory of Acupuncture 132
Modern Theories of Acupuncture 132
Chronic Pain 133
Acupuncture for Chronic Pain/Fibromyalgia 134
How Does Acupuncture Work? 134
Fibromyalgia 135
An Acupuncture Treatment 136
Advantages of Acupuncture 137

CHAPTER **11**   **Visual Problems Concurrent**
with Fibromyalgia 141
Randy Houdek, OD

Eye Problems Directly Related
to Fibromyalgia 142
Complications Secondary to
Treatment Options 150

CHAPTER **12**   **Coming to Terms with Chronic Pain** 153
Peter Ianni, PhD

Fibromyalgia and the Nervous System 153
Treatment 156

CHAPTER 13   ADHD and Fibromyalgia:
             Related Conditions? 165
             Joel L. Young, MD and Judith Redmond, MA

             Surprising Early Findings 167
             Disease-State Impact 168
             ADHD 168
             AFRSC 171
             A Case Study 173
             We Need to Know More 175

CHAPTER 14   A Guy's Perspective: The Other 20%
             of the Fibro Population 179
             Robert S. Leider

CHAPTER 15   Physical Therapy Evaluation and
             Treatment of Fibromyalgia 185
             Loren DeVinney, PT, OMPT

             Brain and Muscle Dysfunction 186
             Special Challenges in Managing Fibromyalgia . . . 187
             Developing a Treatment Plan 187
             Plan of Care 189
             Choosing a Muscle Therapist 195
             Patient Education 195
             The Phases of Physical Therapy 196

CHAPTER 16   Posture/Body Mechanic Training 201
             Loren DeVinney, PT, OMPT

             Proper Posture 202
             Evaluation of Posture 206
             Poor Posture Corrections 207
             Posture Exercises 207
             Body Mechanics 209
             Ergonomics 210
             Conclusion 212

CHAPTER **17**   **Self-Management Techniques** **213**
Sharon Ostalecki, PhD

Learning 215
Journaling 215
Saying "No" 216
Delegating 217
Prioritizing 218
Stress Reduction 219
Support Groups 220
The Basics Summarized 220

CHAPTER **18**   **Healing Through Yoga** **223**
Sarah Bates, OTR, RYT

How and Why Yoga Helps
    Relieve Fibromyalgia 224
Practicing Yoga 225
Attending Yoga Classes 230
For People Experiencing Severe Flare-ups
    or New to Yoga 230
For People Experiencing Moderate
    Flare-ups, Recovering from Severe
    Flare-ups, Stable with Some Symptoms,
    or with Some Yoga Experience 231
For Endurance 231
For People in Remission—Either
    Symptom-Free or Close to It 232

CHAPTER **19**   **Nutrition and Healing** **233**
Sharon Ostalecki, PhD

Disease and Nutrition 234
Hypoglycemia 236
Diet 237
Fuel Efficiency 242
Food Sensitivities 243
A Final Note 248

CHAPTER **20**　**Journey to Motherhood** 249
Gina Hutter

CHAPTER **21**　**Importance of Foot and Ankle Alignment
in Fibromyalgia** 263
Ernst Bastian, CO

Common Foot Problems in
Fibromyalgia Patients 264
Orthotics 268
Shoes 270

CHAPTER **22**　**Behaviorally Reconnecting Mind and Body** ..273
Donald Moss, PhD

The Signs and Symptoms of Fibromyalgia 274
Mechanisms of Fibromyalgia Addressed by
Mind–Body Therapies 275
Precipitating Factors or Events Leading to
the Onset of Fibromyalgia 277
Mind–Body Therapy Approaches
for Fibromyalgia 278
How Can You Benefit? 284
Resources 286

CHAPTER **23**　**Did You Get the License Number of
the Truck That Hit Me?** 289
Jenny Melkvik

Resources 297

Glossary 305

Index 317

Preface

Sharon Ostalecki, PhD

Fibromyalgia (FM) is a chronic pain illness characterized by widespread musculoskeletal aches, pain, and stiffness, soft tissue tenderness, general fatigue, and sleep disturbances. The most common sites of pain include the neck, back, shoulders, pelvic girdle, and hands, but any body part can be affected. Fibromyalgia patients experience a range of symptoms of varying intensities that wax and wane over time.[1]

In the fall of 1991, a Detroit radio show asked me to discuss my experience of living with fibromyalgia. The show generated numerous call-ins, and was well received by listeners. I was asked to return. This time, the physician treating my fibromyalgia (a fibromyalgia and chronic pain specialist) participated in the show. This program, too, went over well. Soon I was being asked to speak at support groups on various topics related to fibromyalgia. Everywhere, I emphasized the importance of developing self-management skills, because my own experience had convinced me of their potential to lessen the symptoms of the disease. I detailed how modifying one's diet might help control the pain of fibromyalgia, but the topic on which I weighed-in most heavily was what I had learned about the *patient's* role in healing.

Over time, word of mouth about my two-pronged approach to nailing fibromyalgia spread. More and more frequently, I was asked to share my experience as a fibromyalgia patient and how it was complemented by my knowledge as a PhD in nutrition.

It became clear to me that whenever and wherever I spoke about fibromyalgia, I had to deal with the topic of frustration—coming from two directions. I addressed the difficult reality that physicians are often frustrated by our multiple complaints and poor prognoses. I talked about how their frustration affected their ability to treat us in an open-minded and optimistic way. I said that it might even discourage them from trying every possible mode of relief, however recent the confirmation that it might be helping other fibromyalgia patients. Then I spoke about the second frustration that got in the way of us getting the best treatment available. I meant our frustration at the difficulty of finding a physician with both the knowledge and temperament to work with us productively. I was becoming increasingly aware of the different shapes fibromyalgia takes and the different ways it affects sufferers. So I knew that, for a physician to treat fibromyalgia productively, he or she would (a) have to keep in mind that each fibromyalgia patient arrives with his or her own particular symptoms, and (b) be willing to work out needed variations of the most successful treatment regimen.

To my surprise—and it was certainly a happy one—every speaking occasion became a learning occasion for me. I paid careful attention to the questions asked and the opinions offered by my audience, and these enriched my own cache of knowledge. In fact, I was able to add the experience of other patients to my own.

Thus, each time I shared, my own share of helpful input grew.

Enthusiastically, then, I developed a three-part lecture series focusing, first, on fibromyalgia; second, on nutrition and healing; and third, on women's health issues. For these lectures I once again teamed with Dr. Martin Tamler (my physician and mentor). Through the lecture series, we tried to educate and help as many people as possible with a disease that affects more than 5 million Americans.

Fibromyalgia affects men as well as women; it happens to people of all ages, including children; and ethnically, it plays no favorites.

At the lectures, people often asked, "How can I find a good fibromyalgia doctor?" I offer here the same answer I would give them—or to anyone who asked me: There is no simple answer to that question. But don't let that discourage you. I will share with you right now much of what I learned during my ultimately successful search—information that should help you in your own hunt for the right doctor.

The very first step is to know your goal. Think through the qualities you're looking for in a doctor. In my opinion, the physician should not only treat your disease, but also be willing to teach you about your illness. You should emerge from a visit to your doctor better equipped to deal with your disease than you were when you walked in. This means your physician should take the time to educate you, not only about fibromyalgia, but also about self-management techniques. Yet another set of qualities you need to look for is openness to new ideas and willingness to try out new concepts and procedures. I think a physician should be willing to consider and learn, not dismiss everything unfamiliar as impossible. We need to be treated by a physician who encourages healing, from whatever source it may come. Above all, perhaps, we need a physician who makes us feel we are capable of experiencing healing.

A few more basics relating to the search for a physician should not be overlooked. If your family physician is unfamiliar with fibromyalgia, then it's best to request a referral to someone who specializes in the disorder. Patients with mild to moderate fibromyalgia can be treated by most rheumatologists and physiatrists. Those with severe cases might do better with a pain physician who specializes in treating the more severe forms of the disorder.

I was fortunate to have the financial resources to "doctor shop"— a term heard a lot in the fibromyalgia community. If you are not free to go to any doctor you choose, you would be wise to educate yourself on every aspect of your disease, because you may have to educate your physician. The development over several years of my personal treatment regimen is proof to me that education is the key to greater understanding, acceptance, and successful management for all who live with the disease. Indeed, *education* is synonymous with *empowerment* when it comes to handling a chronic disease like fibromyalgia.

Encouraged by the feedback I received at lectures when I shared some of my personal experiences, and encouraged by how I felt when listeners turned into sharers too, I saw the good that a regular support system might do. Five years ago, with the help of Lynn Lipmann and Loren DeVinney, I started the nonprofit support group

Helping Our Pain and Exhaustion (H.O.P.E.). Our mission is to increase the knowledge and awareness of available help for fibromyalgia and chronic fatigue syndrome.

In March 2005 and 2006 I was chosen to represent Michigan at the National Fibromyalgia Association's Leaders Against Pain Coalition conference. In meeting with involved physicians and patients from around the country, I discovered that we all had a common purpose in participating in the conference. All of us wanted to be as well-prepared as possible to help people mystified by their symptoms to understand that, no matter what shape their fibromyalgia took, it is possible to learn survival techniques to guide them through "the kingdom of the sick." At the conference, I was heartened to find so many others, like me, determined to make fibromyalgia a disease whose physical existence is validated by the whole community of medical professionals, by the media, and by anyone who still thinks it's "all in the mind."

Over the past decade, I've met hundreds of patients and professionals dealing with this illness. The more people I've spoken with, the more profoundly I've understood that there are many, many pieces to this puzzle called fibromyalgia. The patient and physician working as a team must put together the pieces of the puzzle so that a clear picture emerges.

There is currently no cure for fibromyalgia, and living with fibromyalgia is never simple, but with skilled and understanding help, we can diminish the power of fibromyalgia over our lives. With increasing frequency, new research, new information, and new medications are available or at least visible on the horizon. Physicians' knowledge and attitudes on fibromyalgia are expanding. Given how difficult it has been—and still can be—to find a doctor to treat fibromyalgia, I have been encouraged to learn at lectures and through emails that more and more physicians are coming to believe their patients—and to believe in their ability to get better. It's that growth that not only makes doctors increasingly willing to treat our disorder, but also empowers us to ask for, and receive, the most up-to-date help.

The book you're holding is a valuable tool in learning what you need to know about fibromyalgia. Throughout the process of com-

piling it, I focused on making it a reliable guide for multidisciplinary treatment—a group of treatments proven to work together—to
help those struggling with the symptoms of fibromyalgia. Finding
the right combination of treatments for oneself has a huge benefit: It
makes us feel that we are capable of experiencing lives where pain is
not a constant.

My talks, my travels through the medical maze, what didn't help
me and what did—I have gathered everything that often difficult
adventure taught me and included it in this book. In addition, I
have culled information from carefully selected top professionals to
enrich this resource for patients, families, and friends of those living
with fibromyalgia.

I have also capitalized on my good fortune in becoming
acquainted with many medical professionals who have a helpful outlook on the treatment of fibromyalgia. The result is the information
in this book on all the subjects that concern us, written by thought-
fully chosen experts.

Last, but by no means least, I have included essays by other
patients with the disease, who have been willing to share their stories here.

The most important part of my job was to be an honest broker:
to offer a wide range of opinions from responsible sources. Every
chapter in this book is filled with easy-to-understand advice as well
as answers to many of the questions most often asked by patients.
Most patients treated with a multidisciplinary approach are able to
continue or resume their work lives, to feel physically better and in a
better frame of mind, to participate in activities with family and
friends—in short, to live remarkably normal lives.

From the outset, my goal has been to make this resource for
patients, families, and friends of those living with fibromyalgia
honest and helpful—and, most of all, a book that communicates the
reality of hope.

There *is* hope.

1. National Fibromyalgia Association. http://www.fmaware.org/fminfo/
    brochure.htm#whatIsFibromyalgia.

Contributors

Badr, M. Safwan, MD
Associate Chairman, Department of Internal Medicine
Professor and Chief
Division of Pulmonary, Critical Care and Sleep Medicine
Harper University Hospital
Detroit, Michigan

Bates, Sarah, OTR, RYT
Registered Occupational Therapist
Registered Yoga Teacher
Mountain Center, California

Bastian, Ernst, CO
American Board Certified Orthotist
Wolverine Orthotics, Inc.
Novi, Michigan

DeVinney, Loren, PT, OMPT
Orthopedic Manual Physical Therapist
Clinical Instructor, Oakland University
Private Practice
West Bloomfield, Michigan

Dobritt, Dennis, DO
Pain Management Specialist
American Board of Pain Medicine
Tri-County Pain Consultants
Royal Oak, Michigan
Providence Hospital
Southfield, Michigan

Elkiss, Mitchell, DO
Neurologist
Fellow, American Academy of Neurology
Fellow, American Academy of Medical Acupuncture
Providence Hospital
Farmington Hills, Michigan

Houdek, Randy, OD
Optometrist
Private Practice
Westland, Michigan

Ianni, Peter, PhD
Pain Psychologist
Diplomate, American Academy of Pain Management
Fellow, Biofeedback Certification Institute of America
Private Practice
Farmington Hills, Michigan

Kaspo, Ghabi, DDS
Diplomate Board of Orofacial Pain
Diplomate, Board of the American Dental Sleep Medicine
Private Practice
Troy, Michigan

Meerschaert, Joseph, MD
Board Certified Physiatrist
Diplomate, American Academy of Pain Management
Diplomate, American Board of Pain Medicine
Troy, Michigan

Moss, Donald, PhD
Clinical Psychologist
Integrative Health Studies
Saybrook Graduate School
San Francisco, California

Ostalecki, Sharon, PhD
Nutritionist
Private Practice
Novi, Michigan

Paul, Sander J., MD
Diplomate, American Board of Internal Medicine (ABIM)
Diplomate, ABIM Subspecialty of Endocrinology & Metabolism
Member, Endocrine Society
William Beaumont Hospital
Royal Oak, Michigan
William Beaumont Hospital
Troy, Michigan

Palsson, Olafur S., PsyD
Clinical Psychologist
Associate Professor
Division of Gastroenterology and Hepatology
Department of Medicine
University of North Carolina at Chapel Hill
Chapel Hill, North Carolina

Redmond, Judith, MA
Rochester Center for Behavioral Medicine
Rochester Hills, Michigan

Salloum, Anan, MD
Harper University Hospital
Detroit, Michigan

Schad, Randy, RPh
Registered Pharmacist
Clinical Pharmacist
Detroit Veterans Hospital
Detroit, Michigan

Young, Joel L., MD
American Board of Psychiatry and Neurology
Diplomate, American Board of Adolescent Psychiatry
William Beaumont Hospital
Royal Oak, Michigan

Editor's Biography

Dr. Sharon Ostalecki is the founder and president of Helping Our Pain & Exhaustion. H.O.P.E. is a 501(c)3 nonprofit organization whose mission is to enhance knowledge and awareness of fibromyalgia through educational programs in order to educate families, friends, the public, the media, and the medical community.

Dr. Ostalecki graduated from Eastern Michigan University with a BS in science and a master's in physical science. She holds a PhD in nutrition and specializes in fibromyalgia and chronic fatigue. Her practice is in Novi, Michigan.

For the past 7 years, Dr. Ostalecki has lectured internationally, and has written and published articles on fibromyalgia. She is the Michigan Representative for the National Fibromyalgia Association and an active member of the Leaders Against Pain Coalition. As an active advocate for Fibromyalgia awareness/chronic pain she promotes the Annual Fibromyalgia Awareness Day Proclamation Program. Numerous Michigan mayors and other elected officials have declared "Fibromyalgia Awareness Day" in their jurisdictions. H.O.P.E. has been active in legislative lobbying to raise research funding, FM awareness, and improved patient protection under state and federal laws.

For the past 15 years she has lived with fibromyalgia, and brings her personal insights into her lectures and clinical practice.

CHAPTER

1

Fibromyalgia

Joseph Meerschaert, MD

Peter Ianni, PhD

Many people suffer from chronic, widespread pain. According to the American College of Rheumatology (ACR), about 16% of females and 9% of males report it.[1,2]

Chronic pain is pain that has lasted at least 6 months. *Widespread pain* is pain that arises from many different body structures, which may include joints, spinal discs, muscles, nerves, blood vessels, or organs. The incidence of muscle pain is hard to pinpoint, but most believe it a significant component of chronic widespread pain in most patients.[3]

Understanding Fibromyalgia

Chronic, widespread muscle pain is the hallmark of fibromyalgia (FM). We don't yet know what causes it, but here are some factors implicated in the development of the disease.

For one thing, sustained, intense pain anywhere in the body often triggers reflex muscle contractions in the area, causing pain in those muscles, too.[4] In addition, some people have a deficiency in the body's anti-inflammatory system that causes inflammation to last longer than normal.[5,6]

Moreover, in patients with chronic pain[7,8] we also find the following phenomena:

- *A disruption in the serotonergic inhibitory brainstem pathways, causing widespread allodynia.* The serotonergic inhibitory brainstem pathways are nerve pathways that keep pain from reaching the pain-sensing part of the brain. They keep us from experiencing normal sensations as painful. Hence, disruption of these pathways causes widespread allodynia, a condition in which sensations not normally painful become painful.
- *A defect in the brain's ability to habituate to repetitive stimuli.*[9] When we say that the brain "habituates" to repetitive stimuli, we mean that it becomes less reactive to them, as though it gets used to them. When the stimuli are pain causing, habituation has a natural pain-killing effect. But in fibromyalgia patients this ability to habituate is lacking.
- *A kindling-like phenomenon such as we see in epilepsy.*[10] Normally, brain cells do not stimulate neighboring brain cells. They tend to fire randomly. However, in conditions like epilepsy, brain cells stimulate neighboring brain cells so that they fire together resulting in a seizure. In epilepsy, the area that initially starts the stimulation is limited to one epileptic focus. After several seizures occur, the new epileptic foci develop; they kindle like small fires, each of which can trigger more seizures. When someone experiences recurrent severe pain, additional brain areas become "hot" and this kindling results in amplification of the pain signal.
- *Changes in the slow-transport system, lowering the threshold of stimulation.*[11] As nerve cells fire excessively, changes occur in their slow-transport system. These changes make them fire at lower thresholds.[11] In other words, they become more sensitive, or irritable.

These neurologic changes have profound consequences for individuals who develop fibromyalgia.

Diagnosis

The symptoms of fibromyalgia are similar to those of systemic inflammatory diseases like rheumatoid arthritis, systemic lupus, erythematosus, and scleroderma. To rule out systemic inflammatory disease, primary-care providers refer patients with widespread pain to a rheumatologist. If no other cause for chronic diffuse muscle pain is found, and if the ACR criteria are met, the diagnosis is fibromyalgia.[1]

Over the past 5 years rheumatologists have reported a significant increase in the number of patients referred to them. This is probably due to increased awareness of fibromyalgia by physicians in the primary care setting, not a recent increase in the incidence of fibromyalgia.

In the United States, the prevalence of fibromyalgia is around 3.4% in females and about 0.5% in males.[12] Prevalence increases with age, reaching 7% of females in people from 60 to 79 years old. Why the rate is higher in females is unclear, but accumulating evidence suggests gender-related genetic predispositions.[13]

Regardless of gender, fibromyalgia may be mild, moderate, or severe.[14]

- Mild fibromyalgia is characterized by mild muscle pain—that is, a pain level of 1, 2, or 3 on a 10-point scale. It is little or no hindrance in everyday functioning. Treatment is often by a primary care practitioner (PCP), who may prescribe a tricyclic antidepressant (Elavil, Sinequan, etc.). Symptoms respond to education, instruction in sleep hygiene, self-directed exercise, and over-the-counter medications.

- Moderate fibromyalgia is characterized by moderate muscle pain—that is, a pain level of 4, 5, or 6 out of 10. It somewhat hinders everyday functioning. Some PCPs with pain management experience can manage moderate fibromyalgia, whereas others refer patients to physical medicine and rehabilitation (PM&R) specialists, also known as physiatrists. Patients with moderate fibromyalgia usually need supervised exercise, usually with a physical therapist. They often need a combination of medicines, including anti-inflammatories, muscle relaxants, anticonvulsants, and selective serotonin reuptake inhibitors (SSRIs) or serotonin and norepinephrine reuptake inhibitors

(SNRIs). Patients with moderately severe fibromyalgia often need prescription analgesics.

• Severe fibromyalgia is characterized by severe muscle pain— that is, a pain level of 7, 8, 9, or 10 out of 10. It greatly hinders everyday functioning. Patients are either unable to work or must frequently call in sick. Some have access to an inpatient multidisciplinary program, but usually a physiatrist or other pain management specialist puts together an individualized program that involves several health care providers specializing in the treatment of severe fibromyalgia. They titrate their treatments to maximize pain relief and functioning while minimizing pain flares.

The American Pain Society's medication guidelines for managing fibromyalgia should be followed to maximize pain relief while minimizing side effects.[15] If you need opioid analgesics (codeine, morphine, etc.) most practitioners refer you to a pain psychologist to assess your addiction risk. They also require you to sign a participation agreement. We have found behavioral pain management prudent, as well, because it reduces the need for excessive opioid dosage escalation.

A physiatrist is a specialist in the diagnosis and nonsurgical treatment of pain. A physiatrist usually employs a team approach to restoring a patient's abilities (rehabilitation) through various means, such as medications, physical/occupational therapies, injections, behavioral interventions, and so forth. Therefore, health care providers in other disciplines are often part of the team. Your team members might include a physical therapist, an orthotist, a sleep physician, a nutritionist, a psychologist, and a yoga therapist, for example.

Our primary goals in treating pain are twofold:

• To increase your functional capacity (i.e., how much you can do)
• To minimize the level of pain and suffering

The Examination

Your physiatrist is a team leader, who begins by performing diagnostic examinations to determine the causes of your pain, and then orders various treatment interventions to address those causes.

The word *fibromyalgia* primarily refers to muscle pain. However, patients with muscle pain can also suffer pain emanating from the bones, joints, tendons, cartilage, blood vessels, nerves, discs, and other structures.

Forms

You will probably be asked to fill out several forms prior to your first appointment, providing the following information:

- History of the pain problems (sudden vs. gradual onset, diagnostic workups, response to surgical and nonsurgical interventions, medication history, etc.)
- Medical history (surgeries, illnesses, injuries, visual or hearing problems, etc.)
- Sleep, exercise, eating, and drinking patterns
- Psychosocial history (education, work/marital/substance use history, etc.)
- Description and location of the pain (via drawings, verbal descriptors, 0–10 pain scale, etc.)
- Symptoms of stress, depression, anxiety, irritability, etc.
- Goals (to return to work/school, to reduce medication intake, to obtain better pain relief, to be able to do more, etc.)

Laboratory Tests

Lab tests rule out various illnesses and assess the functioning of your internal organs. These tests require blood and urine samples to determine such things as your thyroid hormone levels, serotonin levels, insulin-like growth factors (IGF), and inflammation levels. Copies of previous lab tests can be helpful, but we usually repeat these tests to make sure nothing has changed.

Initial Physiatric Examination

First, your physiatrist asks questions, some of which have you elaborate on information you provided in filling out the forms. During this talk, you become acquainted with each other. You find out whether your physiatrist is a good listener, whether he or she relates to you in a way you're comfortable with, and so on. During this initial contact, you form the emotional connection that is the essence of the doctor–patient relationship. Your ability and willingness to relate to one another forms the basis for the give and take essential in charting the course of your recovery.

Doctors who treat fibromyalgia and other chronic pain conditions welcome your active participation in your medical care. They are sensitive to your concerns about side effects and risk. Look for signs that your physiatrist understands that rehabilitation is a complex process requiring numerous trial-and-error interventions, because there will be times that you don't respond well, and you must be able to say so without your doctor feeling criticized. Your unfavorable responses (e.g., increased pain or side effects) are as important in guiding treatment as your favorable ones. Of course, your physiatrist tries to minimize the unfavorable responses.

In addition to checking your reflexes, listening to your heartbeat, taking your blood pressure, and so forth, a physiatrist takes other measurements and makes specific observations. We ask when you were last well. We ask about your sleep, whether you have difficulty falling asleep and staying asleep, whether you snore, whether you feel rested when you wake up, and so forth.

Then we do tests to measure visual, auditory, and other sensory (including pain) functions. Through movement tests we assess the functioning of the brain, nerves, muscles, and joints. We assess your sense of balance, and try to determine whether you have numbness in any part of your body. We measure your muscle strength and range of motion (ROM), as well as the speed and pattern of your gait. We measure the length of your arms and legs and examine your feet for abnormalities. We ask about your daily activities, what worsens the pain and what lessens it. Finally, we palpate your muscles to measure the number and size of your trigger points.

Trigger points can occur anywhere in any muscle. To diagnose fibromyalgia, we must find trigger points present in certain well-defined spots. According to the American College of Rheumatology criteria, you must have trigger points in at least 11 of the 18 areas depicted in Figure 1.1.

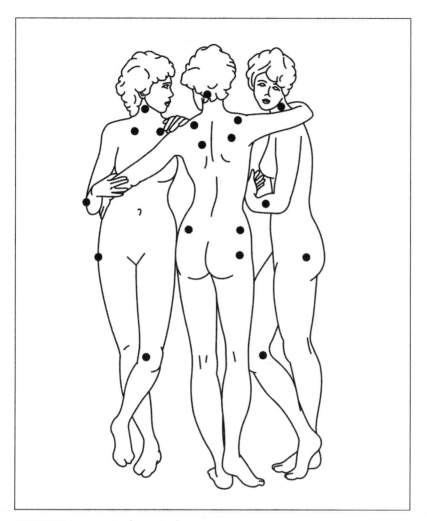

FIGURE 1.1   18 Tender point locations

Additional Diagnostic Tests

Sometimes findings in the initial examination suggest the need for further tests, such as X-rays, CAT scans, MRIs, bone scans, or additional blood tests. We use tests like diagnostic electromyograms and evoked-potential tests to assess the nerve signals traveling from the periphery of the nervous system up the spinal cord to the brain. These tests can provide vital information that should be incorporated into the treatment plan. For example, sometimes patients referred to us with a diagnosis of fibromyalgia have problems with discs or joints in the spine, problems that need to be addressed with injection or surgical procedures.

In addition to the aforementioned tests, we sometimes order a functional capacity evaluation (FCE) to obtain objective measures of how much you are able to lift/carry/push/pull/bend and how long you can stand/sit/work with your arms above your head. These data serve as a baseline measure of your current level of functioning.

The Causes of Pain in FM

Trigger points are painful lumps that develop in taut bands of muscle. They form when a muscle contracts and does not fully release. Their feel can vary from that of a large swollen section of muscle tissue, to small pebbles, to hard spots. When the bands are less taut, there is only muscle tenderness instead of pain. During your examination, the physiatrist presses on the trigger points with 8.8 pounds of pressure, which is just hard enough to lighten the color of his or her fingernail bed.

Human muscle requires ample blood flow to stay healthy, so it has many blood vessels intertwined among the muscle fibers. These blood vessels supply the muscle cells with nutrients and take away waste products. When muscle fibers (which are like long tubes) contract, they shorten, putting pressure on these blood vessels, restricting the flow of blood in them. The restriction of blood flow is a condition known as ischemia. It reduces the supply of nutrients (oxygen and glucose) and causes waste products (acids) to accumulate in the muscle tissue.

When this happens, the walls of the muscle fibers crack and release their fluids, known as prostaglandins, histamine, bradykinin, and neurovasoactive substances.[16] These fluids stimulate pain-sensing nerve fibers in the muscle. Cracks and microscopic tears in muscle (such as occur following exercise) are then repaired in a two-step process.

1. Immune system scavenger cells (in the bloodstream) eat away the muscle fragments that broke off when the cells' walls cracked.
2. Hormones (i.e., growth hormone, corticosteroids, and testosterone), which are used to repair the cracked/torn muscle fibers, flow into the muscle via the bloodstream.

In fibromyalgia, however, the restricted blood flow (and other factors) within the tight muscle prevents this healing process.

There is little focus on central sensitization in mild fibromyalgia. However, we know that those with moderate to severe fibromyalgia suffer from central sensitization. What is central sensitization? It is sensitization within the central nervous system, the brain, and the spinal cord—primarily the brain in this case. This happens because being in constant moderate-to-severe pain causes changes in brain activity. Over time, pain signals arriving at the brain from the pain generators elsewhere in the body (i.e., muscles, joints, and nerves) become amplified as ever-larger areas of the brain are aroused by them.

An elegant experiment using functional MRI (fMRI) testing demonstrates this process.[17] In this experiment we apply 5 pounds of pressure to a person's thumbnail. We ask him or her to rate the pain on a scale of 0–10. We also run an fMRI to see what part of the brain is "lit up" by this stimulus.

People without fibromyalgia report the pain at about 3/10, and their fMRIs show only two brain areas activated. Fibromyalgia patients report the pain at about 8/10, and their fMRIs show greater activation in 13 brain areas. When the normal group's thumbnail pressure is increased to 10 pounds, they report the pain at about 8/10, and their fMRIs show many more brain areas activated.

During pain stimulation, the normal group shows increased activity in the thalamus, a brainstem structure that can reduce the flow of pain information to pain-sensing parts of the brain. In contrast, fibromyalgia patients show reduced activity in the thalamus.

Central sensitization causes amplification of all sensory stimuli—like sounds, visual stimuli, cold, heat, odors, and tastes—not just pain. Consequently, relatively neutral stimuli cause marked discomfort in fibromyalgia patients with central sensitization.

The Treatment Team

As I mentioned previously, a primary care physician can manage mild fibromyalgia. Some patients with moderately severe fibromyalgia, and all patients with severe fibromyalgia, need multidisciplinary or transdisciplinary pain control.

The difference between multidisciplinary and transdisciplinary treatment is in the level of cooperation among team members. In the multidisciplinary approach, each health care provider (e.g., your physical therapist, your orthotist, your sleep physician, and so forth) treats you independently but communicates with other team members. Over time, each team member learns what the others are doing. Eventually, the team's treatments become oriented as a whole.

The team is now a transdisciplinary one in which the health care providers' interventions overlap to fill in and reinforce the goals that characterize the team's treatment orientation. For example, initially, a multidisciplinary team member might tell a patient with severe fibromyalgia to push through the pain, assuming that the pain is mild and the patient just deconditioned. However, once team members begin to identify which patients do poorly when told to push through the pain (i.e., those with moderate-to-severe pain), they make other recommendations like pacing, slowing down, conserving endurance, and resetting priorities. The transdisciplinary approach ensures consistency. You can imagine how confusing it would be for the patient if his or her health care providers gave conflicting instructions because they have no uniform treatment orientation.

Your physiatrist forms several hypotheses about the abnormalities that need to be corrected or addressed. Note that the mere presence of an abnormality doesn't mean that it must be corrected. Even if it does, delaying the treatment of a particular abnormality is often best. The timing of corrective intervention is important to avoid triggering a pain flare. A pain flare can discourage the patient, who has come to the specialist seeking *relief* of pain.

Knowing which corrections to order, which interventions to order, and when to order them is the fruit of the physiatrist's experience with fibromyalgia. Your input is important. Questions are welcome. Learning about the rehabilitation process shapes your understanding of how to get better.

There are many impediments to getting better, because what worked for your mild pain in the past no longer works for the more severe pain you have now. Your physiatrist taps into her or his experience with fibromyalgia patients. In fact, doctors always try to tap into their understanding of what has resulted in recovery versus what has impeded recovery in former patients. Physiatry addresses your pain problems via many different treatments. Although some seem to contribute little to your improvement, the additive effect of several small improvements can be substantial over time.

We consult endocrinologists to rule out endocrine disorders, especially those having to do with thyroid, adrenal, and pituitary hormone systems. Disruption of these systems can cause problems like weight loss or weight gain, fatigue, heart palpitations, and sleep problems.

Physical therapy is the mainstay of physiatric interventions. Physical therapists can address joint, ligament, tendon, nerve, muscle, and other pain generators. They use heat, massage, cold, electrical stimulation, ultrasound, and other therapies. These treatments relieve pain, adjust joints, and correct gait. Physical therapists can also perform interventions to treat balance problems, dizziness, and other symptoms common in fibromyalgia patients.

When pain symptoms permit, the therapist goes on to strength, endurance, and cardiovascular training. Physical therapy fails when you, or the therapist, try to strengthen muscles too quickly. In other words, strength, endurance, and cardiovascular training must be titrated. To do this properly, communication between patient and therapist is critical.

How do we titrate exercise? By altering its intensity, duration, and frequency. Your pain levels may sometimes increase for 12 to 48 hours following a physical therapy session, but the pain should have subsided by the next session. Too much pain means that exercise intensity, duration, and/or frequency must be reduced. If your pain begins increasing without decreasing between physical therapy sessions, you may be experiencing increased muscle contraction, and the exercise can actually cause weakening instead of strengthening.

Many fibromyalgia patients suffer multiple physical therapy failures because their muscles do not relax during physical therapy. If this happens, surface electromyogram (sEMG) biofeedback training can teach you how to make your muscles relax. Once you can relax your muscles, your response to physical therapy can improve.

Massage therapists are often employed to work on releasing the tight bands that contain the trigger points. They can work at a slower pace than physical therapists, and they specialize in various myofascial release techniques.

Orthotists are specialists who make devices to correct structural abnormalities. Sixty percent of the general population has at least a half-inch difference in leg length contributing to their pain problems. Sometimes shoe inserts, used to correct leg-length inequality and gait abnormalities, provide pain relief. When your body leans forward excessively, your lower back and neck muscles must contract to keep you from falling forward. If your body leans backward excessively, your abdominal, pelvic, and upper chest muscles contract to keep you from falling backward. In addition to orthotics, the physiatrist may order braces to support or stabilize the wrist, elbow, knee, or ankle joints. Back braces and neck braces are generally used for only short periods, because you can come to depend on the brace rather than the muscles that should support the body.

Sleep physicians, also known as polysomnographers, may be neurologists, psychiatrists, or pulmonologists.

If you have certain risk factors—like excessive weight or a small neck circumference—your physiatrist will order a sleep study to rule out sleep apnea. If you stop breathing during sleep, you won't cycle properly through the sleep stages, and your blood won't carry enough oxygen to your brain, muscles, and other organs. If you suffer from sleep apnea, you will be given a machine that blows air into your nose to keep your airways open during sleep.

Even if you don't have sleep apnea, take steps to get at least eight hours of sleep per night. Some severe pain patients require 10 or 12 hours. Others do worse if they try to follow good sleep hygiene practices. If severe pain awakens you repeatedly during the night, a nap during the day can reduce pain and fatigue.

Sometimes tooth grinding (bruxism) disturbs sleep. People who grind their teeth may develop temporomandibular dysfunction (TMD commonly referred to as, "TMJ") , which causes jaw, neck, and headache pain.

Dentists who specialize in temporomandibular disorders are skilled at reducing jaw pain. You may be fitted with an oral orthotic or bite splint to wear during the night and, possibly, during the day. Such dentists often work closely with physical therapists who specialize in massage techniques that focus on the chewing muscles.

Nutritionists who understand the needs of fibromyalgia patients are often needed to help you make dietary changes that facilitate healing. Dietary deficiencies can drag you down and contribute to pain. Excess weight can contribute to lower back, knee, foot, and other joint problems. While dieting to lose weight, people often don't get enough protein, which can cause excessive loss of muscle mass. In addition, nausea, fatigue, and pain can sometimes be alleviated by timing meals and drinking more fluids throughout the day. Nutritionists can help you to make dietary changes to address the side effects of medication, and they are on the front lines in monitoring pain patients' responses to supplements.

Rehabilitation/pain psychologists provide many core services in multidisciplinary pain programs. Patients with moderate to severe pain, who have experienced reductions in their functional capacities, undergo multiple grief reactions. Reductions in functional capacities are losses, not unlike losing a loved one, and they trigger feelings that occur in stages: denial, sadness, bargaining with God (when applicable), anger, and acceptance.

Unfortunately, there are cultural prohibitions against feeling sadness over your losses. Yet feeling this sadness is an important part of the mourning process. It is normal to feel sad when you can't keep your house clean. It is normal for a man with chronic pain to feel sad that his wife has to cut the grass. When you feel sad about something, you have hurt feelings that also cause angry feelings. Not allowing yourself to feel the stages of grief prolongs the mourning process.

On the other hand, it is easy for some people to get stuck in the sadness or anger stages, and doing that also interferes with the mourning process. Rehabilitation/pain psychologists help you resolve your grief reactions. They provide strategies for getting the pain (and your life) under better control. They use techniques like biofeedback and cognitive behavioral therapy to teach you how to manage pain better. Psychologists also administer tests to assess suicide and addiction risk and to help your physiatrist understand your emotional needs better. In addition, rehabilitation/pain psychologists provide educational training in understanding your pain generators and how they are being targeted by the interventions your physiatrist has ordered.

Psychiatrists are needed when the pain and depression are in the severe to very severe range. A psychiatrist can also diagnose and treat concurrent conditions such as ADHD. You may be referred to an optometrist or ophthalmologist if you report visual problems. Certain ones are common in fibromyalgia patients, and they can often be addressed via conservative interventions. Visual problems can result in increased head, neck, or facial pain, and trigger points in some of those regions can cause visual problems.

Some yoga therapists are skilled at adapting yoga postures to the limitations caused by chronic pain conditions. Properly done, yoga can reduce pain and strengthen muscles, joints, and ligaments while providing a timeout from the day to practice relaxation.

Acupuncturists are increasingly available specialists, often physicians with specialty training. Acupuncture is, of course, not for anyone with a phobia of needles, but it isn't painful. It appears to reduce central sensitization, and it often helps release muscle contractions, providing immediate analgesia (pain relief) for at least a short time.

If your fibromyalgia is of moderate or severe intensity, you will need long-term management to achieve your goals. You and your physiatrist will choose when to try or retry an intervention. For example, severe-fibromyalgia patients often have multiple courses of physical therapy, during which they quickly plateau due to increased pain.

A Final Word

Periodically review and discuss with your health care providers any changes in your treatment goals, life circumstances, and so forth.

Someday we will better understand the genetic determiners underlying the neurologic, autonomic, and rheumatologic abnormalities that contribute to fibromyalgia. This knowledge may allow the development of gene technologies (like RNA repair) aimed at treating these abnormalities. Each new treatment intervention will alleviate the symptoms of subgroups of fibromyalgia patients, since it appears that fibromyalgia can develop due to the malfunction of different body systems (e.g., the neurologic, immunologic, or autonomic system).

In the meantime, we health care providers do our part by medically addressing the symptoms using the most advanced methods available today. It is your part to do what you can.

References

1. Wolfe F, Smythe HA, Yunus MB, et al. The American College of Rheumatology 1990 criteria for the classification of fibromyalgia. *Arthritis Rheum.* 1990;33:160-172.

2. McBeth J. The epidemiology of chronic widespread pain and fibromyalgia. In: Wallace DJ, Clauw DJ, eds. *Fibromyalgia and Other Central Pain Syndromes.* Philadelphia: Lippincott, Williams & Wilkins; 2005:17-28.

3. Clauw DJ. The taxonomy of chronic pain: moving toward more mechanistic classifications. In: Wallace DJ, Clauw DJ, eds. *Fibromyalgia and Other Central Pain Syndromes.* Philadelphia: Lippincott, Williams & Wilkins; 2005:9-16.

4. Giambardino MA, Affaitati G, Lerza R, Delaurentis S. Neurophysiological basis of visceral pain. *J Musculoskeletal Pain.* 2002;10:151-163.

5. Hallegua DS. Fibromyalgia in inflammatory and endocrine disorders. In: Wallace DJ Clauw DJ, eds. *Fibromyalgia and Other Central Pain Syndromes.* Philadelphia: Lippincott, Williams & Wilkins; 2005:187-195.

6. Uceyler N, Valenza R, Stock M, Schedel R, Sprotte G, Sommer C. Reduced levels of anti-inflammatory cytokines in patients with chronic widespread pain. *Arthritis Rheum.* 2006;54:2656-2664.

7. Mountz JM, Bradley LA, Modell JG, Clauw DJ. Fibromyalgia in women. Abnormalities of regional cerebral blood flow in the thalamus and caudate nucleus are associated with low pain threshold levels. *Arthritis Rheum.* 1995;38:926-938.

8. Yunus MB. The concept of central sensitivity syndromes. In: Wallace DJ, Clauw DJ, eds. *Fibromyalgia and Other Central Pain Syndromes.* Philadelphia: Lippincott, Williams & Wilkins; 2005:29-44.

9. Staud R. The neurobiology of chronic musculoskeletal pain (including chronic regional pain). In: Wallace D, Clauw DJ, eds. *Fibromyalgia and Other Central Pain Syndromes.* Philadelphia: Lippincott, Williams & Wilkins; 2005:45-62.

10. Rome HP Jr., Rome JD. Limbically augmented pain syndrome (LAPS): kindling, corticolimbic sensitization and the convergence of affective and sensory symptoms in chronic pain disorders. *Pain Medicine.* 2000;1:7-23.

11. Kandel E. From metapsychology to molecular biology: explorations into the nature of anxiety. *Amer J of Psychiatry.* 1983;140:1277-1293.

12. Lawrence RC, Helmick CG, Arnett FC, Clauw DJ. Estimates of the prevalence of arthritis and selected musculoskeletal disorders in the United States. *Arthritis Rheum.* 1998;41:778-799.

13. Arnold LM, Hudson JI, Hess EV, Clauw DJ. Family study of fibromyalgia. *Arthritis Rheum.* 2004;50:944-952.

14. McCain G. A clinical overview of fibromyalgia syndrome. *J Musculoskeletal Pain.* 1996;4:9-34.

15. Henrikson KG. Chronic muscular pain: aetiology and pathogenesis. *Ballieres Clin Rheumatol.* 1994;8:703-719.

16. Sprott H. Muscles and peripheral abnormalities in fibromyalgia. In: Wallace DJ, Clauw DJ, eds. *Fibromyalgia and Other Central Pain Syndromes.* Philadelphia: Lippincott, Williams & Wilkins; 2005:101-114.

17. Gracely RH, Petzke F, Wolf JM, Clauw DJ. Functional MRI evidence of augmented pain processing in fibromyalgia. *Arthritis Rheum.* 2002;46:1333-1343.

2

Fibromyalgia: A Patient's Perspective

Jane Charlton

Jane has a wonderful husband (Rob), a son (Max), and they are expecting a new addition to their family. In her spare time she makes jewelry and enjoys reading. Jane has a great group of friends who provide support and love, and with careful medical management she is able to lead a fulfilling life.

— •◆• —

No, you are not crazy. Your pain and fatigue are real and have a cause.

For me it came to a head one day while I was driving home from work on the expressway and suddenly realized, "Oh my gosh, I'm lost."

I pulled off to the side in amazement. Though I was so tired I could hardly think of anything *but* being tired, getting lost cut through the fog to have an impact on me. Where was I? Had I passed my exit? Nothing looked familiar. I had to think back to what I last remembered. I had just left work, hadn't I?

And the little voice in my head kept saying, "I am *so* tired." I broke down and cried, but there was no relief in it, so but a moment later I was saying to myself, "I don't think I've gone far enough" as I pulled back onto the expressway.

Soon, I was crying again. "Maybe I should just run my car into that wall. Then I'd get some *sleep*!" No, I wasn't serious. I was just being sarcastic with myself. All I wanted was to be *myself again*!

I stopped driving that day for over a year. I was 28 years old and had been married for about a year.

That's how overwhelming the pain and fatigue of fibromyalgia can become if it spirals out of control. It can cost you your job. I couldn't keep up with mine. And this was a new job, one I took because it required fewer hours, had fewer deadlines, and involved a shorter commute. Yet I was still so fatigued I would sit in the bathroom with my head against the wall, praying for the strength to make it to lunch. During lunch, I would grab a quick bite to eat and then put two chairs together for a nap so I could begin the afternoon. Then back to the bathroom I'd go to pray that I could make it until my husband picked me up at five. What a life!

That was me then. Before, I had always been an active person. I loved to walk, swim, and spend time with family and friends. Now I just existed.

I couldn't believe it. I don't know what I would have done if my husband hadn't been so supportive. My symptoms continued to spiral, and I had to leave my job, because I just couldn't keep up and was going to get fired if I didn't leave.

I tried working out of my home. Since I developed training courses, a computer, fax, and phone were all I needed. But I continued to get worse. Although I was sleeping as much as I could, I couldn't recharge. I felt drained; just getting out of bed was exhausting. My body felt like it was made of cement. I didn't know what to do. I was losing myself to this pain and fatigue and *nothing* I did seemed to make a difference.

I had been seeing a new physical medicine doctor, who was trying very hard to help me. An office visit consisted of my sitting in the exam room crying, "What is wrong with me? Why can't I do anything? I can't think, I get lost when I drive." He told me to go to the emergency room if I got worse.

I think I was at the hospital within a week. Admission put me on the road to getting better, a returning to my former self. I would love to use the word *recovery* in that last sentence, but fibromyalgia isn't an illness from which you recover. It is a chronic illness that you must learn to manage.

It can be managed; I am living proof.

How did I get here? I was a 28-year-old educated woman who had turned into a shell of my former self. Less than a year before, I held a good job, took a graduate class, and hiked seven miles with my husband on our honeymoon. Before that, I had graduated from college, lived on my own in the Chicago area, and developed training courses for many *Fortune* 500 companies.

Now I was scared to be alone and cried whenever my husband left for work. I couldn't remember my parents' phone number or whether I'd taken my medication. The simplest decisions overwhelmed me. I hadn't the stamina to stand long enough to take a shower, or to sit long enough to go to church.

How did this happen? It was a long, long road to this point. A typical one that may serve as a helpful example to you.

I was an athletic child and teen. I played basketball and swam competitively. I loved to dance and sang in the church choir. I played the bassoon in the symphonic band and a mellophone in the marching band. I biked and walked; I was always on the go.

At fourteen, I began to experience shoulder and neck pain with numbness in my left arm and hand. At sixteen, I was referred to a thoracic specialist in the metropolitan Detroit area. He prescribed exercises for thoracic outlet syndrome—compression of nerves and blood vessels passing through a space between parts of the shoulder blade and collar bone, causing symptoms in the neck, shoulder, and arm.

During the winter when I was sixteen, I injured my left shoulder in swimming practice. This was a very hard time for me. The pain never went away, and the emotional trauma was very difficult. I was a sixteen-year-old girl who could not tie my shoes, dry my hair, or go to the bathroom alone. I had to give up swimming, and my job as a lifeguard and swimming coach. I had to change my class schedule, because I could no longer play music or type.

The fatigue started the year after surgery to remove my top left rib (to relieve the symptoms of thoracic outlet syndrome). I would have days of numbing fatigue. That shouldn't happen to an 18-year-old. As I went on to college, the thoracic-outlet pain in my arm lessened, but the pain in the rest of my body increased, especially in my legs. I didn't understand the pain and fatigue. I didn't understand why I lacked the stamina to do what I'd been able to do before, or why I couldn't keep up with my college classmates' active lives. Nevertheless, I was determined to try to keep up with them.

The pain in my legs got worse through my college years. I prowled the dormitory halls trying to walk out the cramps and the feeling of ants crawling under my skin. Darvocet helped, but to be able to sleep, I had to exhaust myself. The next morning my legs and hips would feel like cement, and it seemed to take forever to get out of bed.

During my second year of college, I saw a neurologist who, despite a negative MRI, diagnosed me with multiple sclerosis. My mother and I actually left that appointment *relieved* and *happy*. Why? Because we finally knew what was wrong with me.

Been there? Just getting a diagnosis can be a feat for people with fibromyalgia. All too often, as in my case, it's a wrong diagnosis.

I would have remained that doctor's patient if she hadn't had such a poorly organized office. (Thank God for small things!) My new neurologist repeated the MRIs and did several spinal taps to confirm that I did not have MS. He was sure I had fibrositis, as fibromyalgia was then called. He weaned me from the MS medication and started me on Elavil.

I did not like the Elavil. Though it helped me sleep, I awoke feeling drugged. In addition, I started craving sugar. Never in my life had I wanted straight sugar on a spoon. Needless to say, I started to gain weight. I took the Elavil for a while and started feeling a little better, but I gained 25 pounds. So I stopped the Elavil and lost 20 pounds. Then the pain and fatigue increased, so I went back on the Elavil. This started a vicious cycle.

The neurologist was not sure how to treat me. I never got full relief of my symptoms and I started developing bad coping techniques.

For years during and after college, I fell into a pattern. To sleep I would overexert myself until I crashed. Then I would drag myself from bed each morning, feeling worse than when I went to bed. I would spend the weekend in bed recovering from the workweek. I would lie to my friends and family, telling them I was sick, because my legs and torso felt like concrete that I could not drag out of bed. Then I would catch a virus and really get sick, which caused such a spike in pain and fatigue that it would take me weeks to recover. I continued in this downward spiral until I was 28 years old.

So how did I get better? While I was in the hospital, I was put on intravenous morphine. My pain eased some, and I began to feel like myself again. I also had many tests performed, one of which measured my serotonin level. My doctor found that it was 4. I believe a normal adult's is somewhere around 120. He told me it was no wonder I was a wreck.

Since morphine can lower serotonin, I was put on oral Vicodin and Ultram for pain. I was already taking Desryll, so my dosage was increased, and Zoloft was added. I also started seeing a pain management psychiatrist and a pain management psychologist. I saw the psychiatrist for a short time, but I still see the pain management psychologist—it has been more than 10 years.

My pain management psychologist helped me learn the difference between good pain and bad pain. He helped me learn to structure my days and not overdo. He taught me that if I have five units of energy for the day, why waste four units walking the grocery store? I should use a scooter to get my groceries. By not walking I saved that energy to spend quality time with my husband. I learned not to struggle with pain just to do the dishes. I'd fill the sink with water and dishes, then lie down. After 10 minutes, I'd wash the dishes, fill the sink again, and lie down again. I followed this process until I again had the strength to wash all the dishes. My pain management psychologist also taught me how to recognize my fatigue signals. I had ignored them for so long that I had to relearn them.

On the medical side, I had a lot of physical therapy, some of it in water. Finally, I started getting better. I started walking on my treadmill one minute a day. After a week, I moved up to two minutes. Although I could have walked longer, I never knew when to stop so that I didn't overdo. So I started slow and listened to my body for signals. As I got better, I was taken off the Zoloft. I also cut back, then eliminated, the Vicodin, then the Ultram. It is amazing to think that at one time I was taking eight Vicodin and eight Ultram a day and still having pain. I also took Buspar for a while to reduce anxiety and Ambien to help me sleep.

One of the most crucial elements of this healing process was recognizing the anger I had because I was sick. I felt that I had no control over my life and that my body had betrayed me. My pain management psychologist's help was very important. Through biofeedback I learned to recognize that I was contracting muscles I wasn't using. Doing so adds to muscle pain and fatigue. I learned how to relax those muscles. I learned that I put way too much stress on myself. Because I felt tired and unable to do things like clean or see friends, I would obsess over not having vacuumed or dwell on the thought that going out to dinner and dancing with friends was too much and life was *so* unfair. Over time I learned a new outlook: *Do I really need to vacuum? Will it make that much difference if I don't do it until Saturday? Why don't I meet friends for dinner and then come home? They are my friends; they will understand, or they should.*

I spent so many years trying to keep up with what my friends could physically do that I lost sight of the big picture: Life is to be enjoyed. I learned I had to plan a little more. I plan my days so that I can enjoy them. *What things are most important to complete this week? What is most important for today? Can I hire the neighborhood teenager to help? How can my family help?* Learning to ask for help and learning to say "no" can dramatically increase your enjoyment of life!

Today I still have ups and downs, but they are nothing compared to what I used to go through. Managing a chronic illness is *not* easy. You may feel fine for a while, and then you catch a virus and symptoms increase. But now I have the skills to cope. Yes, I still feel disappointed and angry at times! And I do get frustrated with myself for failing to recognize the signs quicker. But I know how to stop the slide and get my symptoms on more level ground again. Also, new knowledge has led to more aggressive treatment of my inflammation.

When I'm not feeling good, the first thing I do is review my sleep. *Is it restorative? Do I have pain when I awake?* To help maintain symptom control, I often need to rest during the day. I ask myself, *When was the last time I rested during the day?* I then rearrange my days so that I can rest. *How are my pain levels? Do I need to use a Lidoderm patch to help control pain? Am I eating enough protein? Am I drinking enough water? How is my exercise going? Am I overdoing it? When was the last time my thyroid was checked?* I make a point to slow down and notice that the sky is blue and there are children playing. I remind myself how good a hot shower feels. And so on. When I slow down, I can again focus on what I need in order to be happy and to be comfortable with fibromyalgia.

For those of you who are young women like I was: I went on to have a successful pregnancy. I did have many miscarriages. After consulting with an infertility doctor, I used progesterone and baby aspirin during my pregnancy. I was able to carry my son to full term at the age of 35.

So be persistent in finding help. Learn about your illness and keep informed. Medical science is constantly changing. I always say, "If I only knew 10 years ago what I know today. . . ." I'm sure I'll be saying that forever.

CHAPTER

3

Sleep: An Overview

M. Safwan Badr, MD

Anan Salloum, MD

Sleep is a natural, periodic, and reversible behavioral state. While asleep, we are perceptually disengaged from the environment and unresponsive to it. Overwhelming evidence shows that sleep is essential to life.

The Physiology of Sleep

The defining features of sleep include minimal movement, stereotypic posture, reduced responsiveness to stimulation, and of course reversibility (the ability to awaken).

The Function of Sleep

Why do we sleep?[1] Several hypotheses try to answer that question. The first says that sleep restores physiological processes degraded by continued wakefulness. In other words, sleep is required for restoration and recovery. Despite its intuitive appeal, this hypothesis isn't backed by strong evidence that sleep is restorative.

The second hypothesis is that sleep is required for energy conservation. Accordingly, sleep reduces metabolic rate and body temperature. The third hypothesis, the biologic theory, proposes that reduced motor activity during sleep decreases the likelihood of attracting predators during the hours of the day that an animal need not spend actively feeding or in pursuit of food.

The Effects of Sleep Deprivation

Sleep deprivation has important adverse consequences. In fact, animal studies show that total sleep deprivation is fatal to rats. Several predictable changes occur in sleep-deprived animals. They include the following:

- Body temperature changes
- Heat-seeking behavior
- Increased food intake
- Weight loss
- Increased metabolic rate
- Increased level of norepinephrine (a neurotransmitter) in the blood plasma
- Decreased level of thyroxine (principal thyroid hormone) in the blood plasma
- Increased ratio of triiodothyronine to thyroxine (thyroid hormones)
- Increased levels of the enzyme that controls the generation of body heat by brown fat tissue (A dark-colored, mitochondrion-rich adipose tissue in many mammals that generates heat to regulate body temperature, especially in hibernating animals).

Sleep-deprived rats also get ulcerative and dark brown skin lesions; they die within weeks.[2]

Sleep deprivation in humans brings significant risks to the individual and society, such as an increased risk of motor-vehicle and industrial accidents. For example, several industrial catastrophes (like the nuclear event at Chernobyl and the Exxon *Valdez* accident) were due, at least in part, to sleepy operators.

Another example is medical residency training. Sleep restriction or total sleep deprivation is typical during residents' on-call nights.

The effects on daytime performance and patient safety have received increasing attention over the past few years. For example, the Harvard Work Hours, Health, and Safety Group assessed the effect of extended work hours on resident sleep and health as well as patient safety. In a validated nationwide survey, they found that residents who had worked 24 hours or longer were 2.3 times more likely to have a motor vehicle crash following that shift than when they worked less than 24 hours. They also found that interns working a traditional on-call schedule slept 5.8 fewer hours per week, had twice as many attention failures on night duty, made 36% more serious medical errors, and made nearly six times more serious diagnostic errors than when working on a schedule limiting continuous duty to 16 hours.[3,4]

Chronic sleep deprivation is a common feature of modern life in Western societies. Large-scale studies show that chronic sleep deprivation has substantial, dose-related effects. It decreases vigilance and increases your reaction time.[5] It impairs memory.[6] Other cognitive effects include increased mood disturbance,[7] decreased motivation,[8] and decreased driving ability with increased risk of motor vehicle accidents.[9] Sleep deprivation also has negative effects on the immune system.[10] It increases the risk of cardiovascular events.[11] Finally, sleep curtailment may increase appetite and lead to weight gain.

A recent study shows that sleep curtailment in healthy young men is associated with decreased levels of leptin (an appetite suppressing hormone) and increased levels of ghrelin (which signals the body to eat and store fat), as well as increased hunger and appetite.[12] This is an intriguing new finding with significant implications possibly linking sleep loss with the burgeoning obesity epidemic in the United States, Europe, and the United Kingdom. However, this possible link hasn't been confirmed by large scale population studies.

The Stages and Architecture of Normal Human Sleep

Sleep isn't a passive process, a withdrawal of wakefulness. Instead, it's an active state generated by activity in specific regions of the brain. Thus, sleep is a complex process involving different groups of neurons (nerve cells, including brain cells). There is no single unique "sleep center" in the brain; several areas are important in controlling the state of wakefulness and sleep.

We measure the electrical activity of these areas by a test known as an electroencephalogram (EEG), in which electrodes are placed on the scalp (or sometimes on the brain itself) to measure the "brainwave" activity of the brain cells underneath.

There are **two distinct states of sleep**: rapid eye movement (**REM**) sleep and non-rapid eye movement (**NREM**) sleep. NREM sleep is further subdivided into four stages, according to the Rechtschaffen and Kales scoring system (abbreviated as R & K), which has become the standard method for recording and characterizing sleep in humans.

Typically, sleep is measured in epochs (time periods) of 30 seconds. Each epoch is "scored" and assigned a specific sleep stage.

Rapid Eye Movement (REM) Sleep

REM sleep is also known as paradoxical sleep, during which periods of fast EEG activity recur about every 90 minutes. REM sleep is also characterized by:

- A low voltage, mixed-frequency EEG pattern
- An atonic electromyogram, indicating inactivity of anti-gravity muscles
- Rapid eye movements

Although dreaming can occur during both REM and NREM sleep, REM dreams are more vivid. The function of REM sleep remains uncertain, although some data suggest an important role for REM sleep in memory consolidation.[13]

Non-Rapid Eye Movement (NREM) Sleep

As mentioned earlier, this stage is subdivided into several stages:

- *Stage 1 sleep* is the lightest sleep, a transition from wakefulness to deeper sleep
- *Stage 2 sleep* typically accounts for 40% to 50% of sleep.
- *Stage 3 and Stage 4 NREM sleep* are frequently combined and referred to as slow-wave sleep, accounting for about 20% of total sleep time in adults.

The function of NREM sleep is uncertain, although some reports indicate that slow-wave sleep is restorative.

Sleep stages do not occur randomly, but in cycles, each cycle progressing "deeper" within NREM sleep and ending with REM sleep. The first cycle lasts for about 90 minutes; subsequent cycles last longer, as each cycle's respective REM stage extends.

Circadian Rhythm

Circadian rhythms are 24-hour cycles generated by internal biological clocks, or circadian pacemakers. In mammals, the brain's clock is known as the suprachiasmatic nucleus (SCN) of the anterior hypothalamus region. The circadian period in humans synchronizes to the 24-hour day by external influences, mainly light.[14]

Hormonal Changes During Sleep

Many hormones are affected by the sleep–wake cycle. Growth hormone, prolactin, and parathyroid hormone levels increase during sleep, with growth hormone secretion occurring mainly during slow-wave sleep. Thyroid stimulating hormone (TSH) secretion is suppressed during sleep. In contrast, the pineal hormone, melatonin, is secreted primarily during the hours of darkness.

In fact, light suppresses melatonin secretion. Likewise, some drugs can influence the body's levels of melatonin, either by interfering with its production or due to metabolism. Melatonin promotes sleep and contributes to the regulation of the sleep–wake rhythm. Administration of exogenous melatonin in the early evening hours advances the circadian clock (facilitates earlier sleep).

Melatonin has gained popularity as a sleep promoting agent. Some studies suggest that melatonin may be useful in the treatment of delayed sleep phase syndrome, jet lag, work shifts, and insomnia in older people with low endogenous melatonin levels. However, evidence remains limited and inconclusive. A recent meta-analysis showed no evidence that melatonin is effective in treating secondary sleep disorders or sleep disorders accompanying sleep restriction, such as jet lag and shift-work disorder. The FDA doesn't approve melatonin for the treatment of insomnia.[15] Available preparations are sold as nutritional supplements, not as medications.

Sleep Disorders

The second edition of the International Classification of Sleep Disorders (ICSD) lists 85 sleep disorders in eight major categories:

- Insomnias
- Sleep-related breathing disorders
- Hypersomnias not due to a breathing disorder
- Circadian rhythm sleep disorders
- Parasomnias
- Sleep-related movement disorders
- Other sleep disorders

Isolated symptoms, due to adverse effects of drugs, medications, or biological substances.

In this review, we will discuss mainly the first two sleep disorders listed above.

Insomnia

Insomnia is inadequate quality or quantity of sleep, with difficulty initiating or maintaining sleep. Insomnia is associated with non-restorative sleep and complaints of impaired daytime functioning. It is the most common sleep disorder in the United States.

Dyssomnia are primary disorders of sleep. The ICSD classifies insomnia as a dyssomnia, and it is a main symptom in 40 categories of sleep disorders. Insomnia occurs with extrinsic, intrinsic, and circadian rhythm sleep disorders.

Risk Factors

Several physiologic and pathologic conditions are associated with a higher prevalence of insomnia. These include female gender, older age, health status, chronic pain, lower socioeconomic status, marital status (higher prevalence in divorced, separated, or widowed people), and various other behavioral and environmental factors. Insomnia also occurs more frequently with depression and drug or alcohol abuse.

Causes

Many medical, neurological, psychiatric, and primary sleep disorders can cause insomnia (see Table 3.1). We also see more insomnia

TABLE 3.1 Causes of Transient and Short-Term Insomnia (less than 3 months)

A change of sleeping environments
Jet lag
Changes in work shift
Environmental factors
Stressful life events
Acute medical or surgical illnesses—chronic pain
Stimulant medications

in patients with chronic pain. Studies that address the interaction between syndromes that cause chronic pain (like fibromyalgia and irritable bowel syndrome) and sleep remain inconclusive. The most common sleep abnormalities found in patients with chronic pain include:

- Lower sleep efficacy (ratio of total sleep time to time in bed)
- Longer percentage of sleep time in Stage 1, with less in Stages 3 and 4 in some disorders
- Sleep stage shifts—frequent changes in sleep state resulting in "lighter" sleep (e.g., Stage 3 and Stage 4 shift toward Stage 2 or Stage 1).
- Fragmentation of sleep continuity

Common Primary Sleep Disorders Associated with Insomnia

The two main primary sleep disorders associated with insomnia are psycho-physiologic insomnia and circadian rhythm disorders.

Psycho-physiologic insomnia is a chronic insomnia accounting for 15% of insomnia cases. It usually starts in young adulthood as a transient insomnia after a stressful event, and then the insomnia persists secondary to excessive worry about being unable to sleep.[16]

Circadian rhythm disorders include two distinct syndromes: delayed sleep phase syndrome and advanced sleep phase syndrome. In delayed sleep phase syndrome, sleep onset is delayed. The patient has trouble falling asleep and awakening at the desired time. In contrast, in advanced sleep phase syndrome, sleep onset occurs in the early evening, and the patient wakes up too early.[17] Diagnosis is based on sleep logs and normal sleep architecture during a polysomnography (i.e., a sleep study). Table 3.2 lists tips for good sleep.

Evaluation and Management of Insomnia

Clinical evaluation of insomnia requires a complete history and physical examination, including a detailed sleep history, social habits, drugs and alcohol consumption, as well as personal and familial medical and psychiatric history. Physical examination is often negative. Determining your sleep habits requires a detailed sleep diary for 2–4 weeks (see Figure 3.1). A detailed diary is indispensable for formulating a differential diagnosis and a treatment plan. Objective testing in the sleep laboratory is rarely required, unless other sleep disorders are suspected.

There are two kinds of treatment for insomnia: conservative therapies and pharmacologic therapies.

Nonpharmacologic, conservative therapy focuses on cognitive-behavioral therapy (CBT). The mainstay of this approach is to follow proper sleep hygiene guidelines. Other techniques, including stimulus control therapy and relaxation techniques, are also incorporated into the treatment plan.[18] The initial therapy is within the scope of a sleep medicine practice. However, advanced CBT and relaxation techniques require specialized training by clinical psychologists. The effectiveness of CBT has been demonstrated in randomized, controlled trials. However, CBT requires several weeks of dedicated therapy and may not be readily available in all centers.

Pharmacologic therapy is being increasingly used. Many patients use over-the-counter medications like antihistamines. In other cases, sleep specialists treat insomnia with sedating antidepres-

TABLE 3.2 Tips for Good Sleep Hygiene[18]

Avoid caffeinated beverages, alcohol, and tobacco in the evening.
Avoid intense mental activities and vigorous exercise close to bedtime.
Follow a regular sleep–wake schedule.
Avoid forcing sleep and daytime naps.

sants and other medications that sedate as a side effect. However, this approach is not recommended unless patients are receiving appropriate therapy for a specific psychiatric disorder.

Many patients with insomnia report self-medicating with over-the-counter medications or alcohol. Commonly used nonprescription medications include antihistamines, cough syrups, aspirin, and several unregulated dietary supplements. There is no evidence to support the use of such agents in the treatment of insomnia. Likewise, alcohol disrupts sleep, suggesting that the use of alcohol may exacerbate, rather than alleviate, insomnia.

Several pharmacologic agents are available. Most are classed as hypnotics. Several vary in half-life and duration of action. Hypnotics carry the risk of tolerance and dependence, and should be

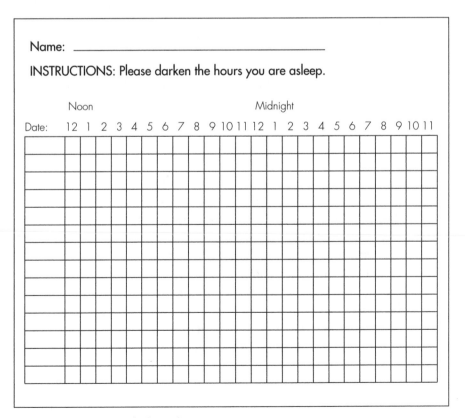

FIGURE 3.1 A 2-week sleep diary.

used for a limited period whenever possible. However, patients with chronic, refractory insomnia often receive pharmacologic therapy for extended periods.

Sleep-Related Breathing Disorders

Abnormal breathing during sleep is an increasingly recognized clinical problem. Patients with lung disease, such as asthma and chronic obstructive airway disease (COPD), may develop periods of even worse oxygenation of the body's tissues during sleep, because of the decreased frequency and depth of breathing during sleep. However, the term *sleep-related breathing disorder* is mostly applied to sleep apnea and hypopnea syndrome.

The sleep state weakens the stimulus to breathe, causing narrowing and increased resistance in the upper airway. This is normal and leads to an increased level of carbon dioxide (measured as PCO_2) in the arteries during sleep. Snoring occurs when upper airway resistance increases significantly, leading to "fluttering" of the soft palate due to turbulent flow. A more pronounced narrowing of the upper airway leads to reduced ventilation of the lungs (hypopnea) or complete cessation of breathing (apnea).

Snoring: More Than a Nuisance

Snoring is an acoustic phenomenon. Usually it happens on inhalation and is caused by fluttering and vibration of the soft tissues of the upper airway. Snoring is common, occurring in about 40% of adults.[19] Clinically, the bed partner, not the patient, is the one to complain about snoring. Although most patients with sleep apnea (discussed in the following section) report snoring, most snorers do not have sleep apnea. Thus, it is important to distinguish primary snoring from snoring as a marker of a more serious disorder such as obstructive sleep apnea (OSA) syndrome.

Snoring may be associated with adverse consequences, even in the absence of sleep apnea. Although the evidence to date is insufficient to conclude that snoring is an independent risk factor for hypertension,[20] some large studies found that nonapneic snoring (i.e., snoring not associated with sleep apnea) was weakly, but independently, associated with hypertension.[21] In addition, snoring may be associated with recurrent episodes of brief arousal from sleep. This is often referred to as the "upper airway resistance syndrome." Whether it is a separate condition is still unclear.

Treatment of snoring depends on the clinical picture. If snoring is part of sleep apnea syndrome, we aim treatment at the primary sleep disorder. Primary snoring can be treated conservatively. However, the distinction between snoring and sleep-related breathing disorder isn't sharp. Snoring falls somewhere between normal physiology and pathology, depending on the accompanying clinical features. Thus, treatment strategies for snoring and mild sleep apnea may be quite similar.

The management plan includes weight loss, smoking cessation, and alcohol avoidance. Not sleeping on your back may also be beneficial in some patients. If nasal obstruction is contributing to snoring, relief of nasal obstruction and appropriate treatment for allergy may be beneficial. Other available treatments, such as mechanical nasal dilators, haven't been rigorously evaluated. We might recommend an oral appliance if the aforementioned treatments don't alleviate snoring.

Obstructive Sleep Apnea Syndrome

Apnea is a Greek word that means "without breath." Physiologically, apnea can be classed into three types: central, obstructive, and mixed.

Central apnea is the cessation of airflow without any respiratory effort to move air into or out of the lungs. Conversely, obstructive apnea is the cessation of airflow for more than 10 seconds with ongoing respiratory effort—as though the patient is trying to breathe. Mixed apnea contains components of both types of apnea.

Obstructive sleep apnea (OSA)/hypopnea syndrome is a clinical condition characterized by repeated episodes of upper airway obstruction. This may manifest as apnea or hypopnea. In apnea, the obstruction is complete; in hypopnea, it is partial.

Sleep apnea/hypopnea syndrome is common in adults. The estimated prevalence of sleep-disordered breathing (defined as an apnea/hypopnea index of more than five events per hour) is 9% for women and 24% for men (in the age range from 30–60 years). When the apnea/hypopnea index is combined with reported sleepiness (i.e., sleep apnea syndrome), 2% of women and 4% of men meet the minimal diagnostic criteria.[19]

The main symptoms reported with obstructive sleep apnea syndrome include:

- Snoring
- Excessive daytime sleepiness
- Witnessed apnea
- Multiple nocturnal arousals

The immediate effects of an apneic episode include hypoxia (deficiency of oxygen in body tissue) and repeated arousals from sleep. The brain arouses from sleep under these conditions to correct the situation by increasing ventilation.

Other immediate consequences of apnea include arrhythmia (heart palpitations) and cardiac ischemia (inadequate blood flow). Repeated episodes of apnea/arousal lead to fragmented sleep, nonrefreshing sleep, and subsequent daytime sleepiness. Therefore, the risk of motor vehicle accidents is higher in patients with sleep apnea than in the general population. In addition, sleep apnea is associated with increased prevalence of high blood pressure,[20] cardiovascular disease,[22] and stroke.[23] In fact, there is extensive evidence that sleep apnea is an independent risk factor for cardiovascular disease and death.

Diagnosing sleep apnea requires monitoring in the sleep laboratory to record sleep and respiration. The test, commonly called a polysomnography (PSG), makes multiple recordings of sleep, respiration, and body position. Sleep states are distinguished by recording an EEG, an electrooculogram (EOG) of the eyeballs, and an electromyogram (EMG) of the chin muscles. Cardiopulmonary monitoring records oxygen saturation of the blood, airflow, respiratory effort, and heart rate (see Figure 3.2). The metric used is the apnea/hypopnea index (AHI), which is the number of apneas and hypopneas per hour of total sleep time. An apnea/hypopnea index of five events per hour of sleep is considered the cutoff for diagnosis of sleep apnea.

Treatment

Treatment options for OSA include conservative approaches similar to those used for snoring. The treatment of choice for sleep apnea is

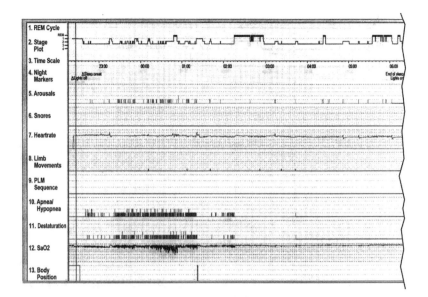

FIGURE 3.2   A polysomnography summary.

positive pressure therapy via a nasal or oral mask. This is because upper airway obstruction can be eliminated by simply increasing the pressure in the upper airway above atmospheric pressure. We do this with nasal positive airway pressure (PAP). The appropriate pressure is determined in the sleep laboratory during polysomnography. PAP is effective in eliminating sleep apnea and improving the natural history of the condition in most patients. Some patients don't stick to this therapy, though. That is mainly because many patients have difficulty tolerating nasal CPAP (Continuous Positive Airway Pressure) due to nasal airway problems, mouth leak, and general discomfort from the mask and headgear.

Additional therapeutic options include oral appliances, mostly in mild cases. These devices function by advancing the mandible and increasing the diameter of the upper airway. Advances in manufacturing oral appliances allow patients to gradually increase the diameter of the airway opening as they get used to the appliance, resulting in successful treatment of more patients. It is important to repeat polysomnography in patients with moderate or severe disease to make sure that oral appliances are effective enough.

The last treatment option is surgical modification of the upper airway, via either soft tissue surgery or skeletal surgery. This approach is used in patients who decline or don't tolerate nasal CPAP therapy and who aren't candidates for oral appliances. In severe cases, bypassing the upper airway with a tracheostomy is the definitive and curative therapy for obstructive sleep apnea.

As you can see, several treatment options are available for obstructive sleep apnea. Nasal CPAP is the treatment of choice, but oral appliances and surgery have distinct roles that are likely to become more defined in the future.

Conclusion

Sleep is essential to life, though the reasons why we sleep are not yet clear. Sleep disorders and sleep-related breathing disorders are common and may have a significant impact on individual and public health. Therefore, attention to sleep is an important component of comprehensive evaluation by health practitioners.

Sleep disorders and sleep-related breathing disorders are especially common among those suffering from chronic pain, like fibromyalgia patients. So, if you suffer from fibromyalgia, make sure any sleeping problems you have are dealt with.

References

1. Horne J. *Why We Sleep.* Oxford, UK: Oxford University Press; 1988.
2. Rechtschaffen A, Bergmann BM. Sleep deprivation in the rat by the disk-over-water method. *Behav Brain Res.* 1995 Jul-Aug;69(1-2):55-63.
3. Harvard Work Hours, Health, and Safety Group: extended work shifts and the risk of motor vehicle crashes among interns. *N Engl J Med.* Jan 13, 2005;352(2):125-134.
4. Lockley SW, Landrigan CP, Barger LK, Czeisler CA. Harvard Work Hours, Health, and Safety Group: when policy meets physiology: the challenge of reducing resident work hours. *Clin Orthop Relat Res.* Aug 2006;449:116-127.
5. Belenky G, Wesensten NJ, Thorne DR, et al. Patterns of performance degradation and restoration during sleep restriction and subsequent recovery: a sleep dose-response study. *J Sleep Res.* Mar 2003;12(1):1-12.

6. Van Dongen HP, Maislin G, Mullington JM, Dinges DF. The cumulative cost of additional wakefulness: dose-response effects on neurobehavioral functions and sleep physiology from chronic sleep restriction and total sleep deprivation. *Sleep.* Mar 15, 2003;26(2):117-126. Erratum in: *Sleep.* Jun 15 2004;27(4):600.
7. Dinges DF, Pack F, Williams K, et al. Cumulative sleepiness, mood disturbance, and psychomotor vigilance performance decrements during a week of sleep restricted to 4-5 hours per night. *Sleep.* 1997;20:267-277.
8. Ewing SB, Balachandran DD, LeBeau L, et al. Subjective and objective indices of sleep loss: effects of chronic partial sleep restriction. *Sleep.* 2002;25:A448.
9. Stutts JC, Wilkins JW, Osberg JS, et al. Driver risk factors for sleep-related crashes. *Accid Anal Prev.* 2003;35:321-331.
10. Spiegel K, Sheridan JF, Van Cauter E. Effect of sleep deprivation on response to immunization. *JAMA.* 2002;288:1471-1472.
11. Ayas NT, White DP, Manson JE, et al. A prospective study of sleep duration and coronary heart disease in women. *Arch Intern Med.* 2003;163:205-209.
12. Hobson J. *Sleep.* New York: Scientific American Library; 1989.
13. Smith C, Wong PTP. Paradoxical sleep increases predict successful learning in a complex operant task. *Behav Neurosci.* 1991;105:282-288.
14. Klein D, Moore R, Reppert S. *Suprachiasmatic Nucleus: The Mind's Clock.* New York: Oxford University Press; 1991.
15. Buscemi N, Vandermeer B, Hooton N, Pandya R, Tjosvold L, Hartling L, et al. Efficacy and safety of exogenous melatonin for secondary sleep disorders and sleep disorders accompanying sleep restriction: meta-analysis. *BMJ.* Feb 18, 2006;332(7538):385-393. Epub Feb 10, 2006.
16. Hauri P, Fisher J. Persistent psychophysiologic (learned) insomnia. *Sleep.* 1986;9(1):38-53.
17. Wagner DR. Disorders of the circadian sleep-wake cycle. *Neurol Clin.* Aug 1996;14(3):651-670.
18. Bootzin RR. Stimulus control treatment for insomnia. Programs and abstracts of the 80th Annual Convention of the American Psychological Association; September 2, 1972; Honolulu, Hawaii.
19. Young T, Palta M, Dempsey J, Skatrud J, Weber S, Badr S. The occurrence of sleep-disordered breathing among middle-aged adults. *N Engl J Med.* Apr 29, 1993;328(17):1230-1235.
20. Nieto FJ, Young TB, Lind BK, Shahar E, Samet JM, Redline S, et al. Association of sleep-disordered breathing, sleep apnea, and hypertension

in a large community-based study. Sleep Heart Health Study. *JAMA.* Apr 12, 2000;283(14):1829-1836.

21. Bixler EO, Vgontzas AN, Lin HM, et al. Association of hypertension and sleep-disordered breathing. *Arch Intern Med.* 2000;160:2289-2295.

22. Marin JM, Carrizo SJ, Vicente E, Agusti AG. Long-term cardiovascular outcomes in men with obstructive sleep apnoea-hypopnoea with or without treatment with continuous positive airway pressure: an observational study. *Lancet.* Mar 19-25, 2005;365(9464):1046–1053.

23. Yaggi HK, Concato J, Kernan WN, Lichtman JH, Brass LM, Mohsenin V. Obstructive sleep apnea as a risk factor for stroke and death. *N Engl J Med.* Nov 10, 2005;353(19):2034-2041.

4

Interventional Treatments for Fibromyalgia and Other Pain Conditions

Dennis W. Dobritt, D.O.

Fibromyalgia is a chronic pain disorder usually described as widespread musculoskeletal aches and pains. It occurs in 2% of the population, with 3–6 million Americans suffering from this condition. Women are by far the most likely to develop the disorder, but men and children get it, too.

In addition to muscle aches and pains, the symptoms of fibromyalgia include tender points, stiffness, soft tissue swelling, muscle spasms, fatigue, sleep disturbances, anxiety, depression, irritable bowel and bladder, headaches, restless legs syndrome, impaired memory and concentration, skin sensitivities, rashes, dry eyes and mouth, ringing in the ears, dizziness, vision problems, Raynaud's syndrome, neurological symptoms, and impaired coordination. These symptoms are also seen in other common medical disorders like diabetes, thyroid problems, spinal disorders, and neurological conditions including neuropathy. Therefore, physicians must rule out these other conditions before diagnosing fibromyalgia.

In 1990 the American College of Rheumatology established criteria for diagnosing fibromyalgia. The first criterion is a history of pain that is widespread in a body region for at least 3 months. The affected body region may be:

- The entire left or right side of the body
- The entire body above or below the waist
- The axial skeleton

Axial skeletal pain is primarily back and neck pain, but the axial skeleton includes all the bones in the head and trunk of the body, including the skull and ribs, as well as the spine.

In addition to widespread pain in one of these body regions, there must be 11 of 18 tender points in specific areas, including the occiput, low cervical, trapezius, supraspinatus, second rib, lateral epicondyle, gluteal, greater trochanter, and knees (see Figure 1.1 in Chapter 1).

The causes of fibromyalgia are unclear. Recent research suggests a genetic predisposition to developing a central nervous system disorder (i.e., a disorder of the brain and spinal cord) that affects the response to severe pain. There also appears to be a problem with a vast network of nerve pathways in the brain, spinal cord, and throughout the body known as the autonomic nervous system.

You might think of the autonomic nervous system as the "automatic" nervous system, the part that controls the body's life support functions, such as breathing, heart rate, blood pressure, and so forth. It regulates hormones and transmitter substances produced by the brain, and some studies show differences in fibromyalgia patients here: They have an increase in substance P, a decrease in serotonin and tryptophan, reduced blood flow to the thalamus (the top of the spinal cord), and reduced function of the hypothalamus-pituitary-adrenal hormone system. The result is amplified pain or sensitivity. The increased pain sensitivity may also cause fibromyalgia patients to feel pain in areas (e.g., discs, joints, and so forth) that were not painful prior to the onset of muscle pain.

For some patients, pain onset is gradual and insidious. However, some fibromyalgia sufferers develop the symptoms following an illness or traumatic injury. This illness or injury may trigger fibromyalgia symptoms in a person genetically predisposed to develop problems with central nervous system processing and/or with autonomic functioning.

Currently, there is no laboratory or radiological test for fibromyalgia. The diagnosis is clinical and based on the patient's history and physical findings, while ruling out any other conditions that might present with the same symptoms.

Many fibromyalgia symptoms also occur in other common pain conditions such as myofascial pain dysfunction syndrome and spinal pain. The treatment for fibromyalgia is symptom management and is discussed in other chapters of this book. This chapter will tell you about pain treatment options that are available for fibromyalgia and for many other common painful conditions that can co-exist with fibromyalgia.

These therapies directly modulate pain by using small needles or tools to deliver medication or treatment to the site of pain generation. The treatments that will be discussed are:

- Trigger point injections
- Nerve blocks
- Spinal injections
- Cryolesioning
- Radiofrequency lesioning
- Intervertebral disc procedures
- Advanced interventional therapies

Trigger Point Injections

Trigger points are discrete, focal areas of taut muscle bands. They are highly irritable, and when compressed can produce referred pain and tenderness, muscular dysfunction, and autonomic nervous system symptoms. Contrast this to tender points, which produce pain only when palpated and do not refer pain so that you feel it in other parts of the body.

Trigger points cause a common painful disorder known as myofascial pain dysfunction syndrome. This disorder is different from fibromyalgia syndrome, which involves multiple tender spots or tender points. These pain syndromes often occur together and may interact with one another, producing both tender points and trigger points. Trigger points are classified as active, latent, or satellite, and are well described in Dr. Janet Travell's classic textbook, *Myofascial Pain and Dysfunction: The Trigger Point Manual.*

An active trigger point causes pain at rest, is tender to palpation, and has a referred pain pattern similar to the patient's pain complaint. Referred pain is an important characteristic of a trigger point and differentiates it from a tender point, which is associated with pain at the site of palpation only. A latent trigger point does not cause pain at rest. The presenting symptom may not be pain at all, but rather a reduced range of muscle motion or weakness. The patient may become aware of pain originating from a latent trigger point only when pressure is directly applied to the area. Satellite trigger points occur in muscle groups distant to the site of pain, and may be due to compensation or overuse of the affected muscle.

Trigger points are associated with a "twitch response." The twitch response is elicited when firm pressure is applied with the fingers perpendicular to the trigger point in a snapping manner, or when a needle is injected directly into the trigger point. Trigger points that do not respond to more conservative therapies, such as massage, physical therapy, or spray and stretch, are treated by injecting them with a small needle using local anesthetic with or without a corticosteroid. Trigger point injections can be repeated several times to facilitate an exercise program or physical therapy.

Figure 4.1 demonstrates a trigger point injection.

Nerve Blocks

Nerve blocks are injections to treat or alleviate pain in a region by delivering medication to the nerve(s) that blocks the flow of pain

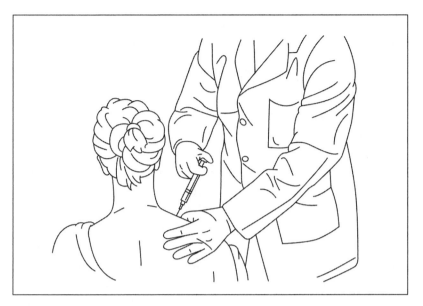

FIGURE 4.1   Trigger point injection

signals. A local anesthetic, sometimes used with corticosteroids, is injected near a nerve or group of nerves. Nerve blocks provide immediate pain relief by temporarily numbing the nerve. If done repeatedly or in series, they may produce long-lasting results. The corticosteroid medication sometimes used is similar to chemicals naturally produced by the body's adrenal glands (methylprednisolone or triamcinolone). It reduces nerve inflammation caused by pressure from surrounding joints, discs, muscles, or scar tissue. Commonly performed nerve blocks include the occipital nerve block, peripheral nerve blocks, and sympathetic nerve blocks.

Headaches occur frequently in fibromyalgia patients. The headaches may be:

- Vascular headaches, due to dilation of blood vessels in the skull
- Muscle-tension headaches
- Occipital neuralgia (pain in the nerves in the lower back part of the skull)

For example, migraine headaches are vascular headaches. Muscle-tension headaches are due to problems in the cervical spine, like cervicogenic headaches. The greater occipital nerves run from the top of the back of the head down to the base of the skull. There they travel through muscles that can compress them, causing them to become inflamed, resulting in occipital neuralgia.

An occipital nerve block is the most common nerve block performed for headache pain. The greater occipital nerve is close to the surface and passes through muscle tissue below the base of the skull about 3 to 4 centimeters to either side of the midline. We can block the nerve by injecting 3 to 5 cubic centimeters of local anesthetic with corticosteroids. The procedure is safe, requires but a small gauge needle, and can be performed in the physician's office without special equipment. We think this block works by interrupting the pain reflex to let the muscles relax and by the anti-inflammatory effects of the corticosteroids. Side effects and complications are rare.

A physician with the skill, training, and proper equipment can perform nerve blocks on nearly all the peripheral nerves. Many peripheral nerve blocks require special training and X-ray guidance using fluoroscopy (live X-ray), but most physicians who have completed specialty training in pain management do have the necessary skills to perform these procedures.

If a fibromyalgia patient has considerable muscle pain and spasm to an entire body region, such as an arm or a leg, then a peripheral nerve block to that region may provide immediate short-term pain relief by temporarily interrupting the pain reflex and facilitating physical therapy interventions.

Nerve blocks to the autonomic or sympathetic nervous system are often helpful in alleviating extremity pain due to autonomic dysfunction. Other causes such as trigger points, nerve injury, vascular disease, and reflex sympathetic dystrophy may result in excessive activation of the sympathetic division of the autonomic nervous system. This causes excessive blood vessel constriction, sweat gland stimulation, and muscle contraction in the affected limb. Injecting local anesthetic near the sympathetic ganglia (clusters of nerve-cell connections) can interrupt this pain.

The sympathetic ganglion of the arm is called the stellate ganglion. The left and right stellate ganglia are in the middle of the neck at its base, on either side of the windpipe. There is one stellate ganglion for each arm. We can block it by injecting 5 to 10 cubic centimeters of dilute local anesthetic. Fluoroscopy may be necessary to guide the physician in inserting the needle. The block usually lasts for several hours but may last for days or weeks. We often do a series of injections for long-term relief.

A stellate ganglion block is considered a safe procedure if done by properly trained physicians. Serious side effects and complications can occur, but are rare. The potential risks and complications include bleeding, infection, spinal block, epidural block, and injection into blood vessels or surrounding organs.

Injecting the lumbar (lower back) paravertebral sympathetic ganglion can block the autonomic nervous system of the leg. This technique is analogous to the one just described for the arm. The lumbar paravertebral sympathetic ganglia lie alongside the second through fifth lumbar vertebrae, one on each side. We block the ganglion by injecting 10 to 15 cubic centimeters of local anesthetic at two points next to the second or third lumbar vertebra on the same side as the painful limb. This procedure requires special training and X-ray guidance using fluoroscopy. As with the stellate ganglion block, this block generally lasts for several hours but may last for several days or weeks. We often do a series of injections over several weeks if the patient reports significant relief with the diagnostic block.

The potential risks and complications include bleeding, infection, spinal block, epidural block, spinal headache, and injection into blood vessels and surrounding organs. Fortunately, serious side effects and complications are rare when performed by properly trained physicians.

Spinal Injections

Low back pain is one of the most common pain conditions experienced by Americans. At some time in their life, 80% will experience low back pain severe enough to seek medical attention. At any given time, over 30 million Americans suffer from low back pain. Neck pain is also thought to be a very common condition. It is not surprising, then, that people with fibromyalgia are likely to experience spinal pain at the same time that they are experiencing muscle pain and other types of pain.

Unlike other skeletal pain, such as strains or sprains, back pain isn't caused only by muscles, tendons, and ligaments. There are other structures in the spine that generate pain. These include the discs, vertebrae (bones of the spine), nerve roots, facet joints (where the sides of the vertebrae meet), and sacroiliac joints (where the lowest part of the spine connects to the pelvis).

The spinal column is a complex structure. There are 7 cervical (neck), 12 thoracic (mid-spine), 5 lumbar (lower spine), 5 sacral (lowest spine), and 5 coccygeal (tailbone) vertebrae for a total of 34. The sacral and coccygeal vertebrae are fused and are essentially a single vertebra. There is an intervertebral disc between each pair of vertebrae, which serves as a shock absorber. Each vertebra has two facet joints that allow the different directions of motion in the spinal column.

Adding up all the possibilities, it is no wonder why spine pain is so common.

At first glance, it seems a daunting task to sort out all the possible pain generators in the spine. No diagnostic test tells us what causes back pain. X-rays and MRIs show only anatomical abnormalities that *may* be the source of pain.

But fortunately we know ahead of time that 40% of lower back pain is due to discs, 40% to facet joints, and 15% to the sacroiliac joints. The same holds true for the cervical and thoracic spine, except there are no sacroiliac joints. The analogous structure in the cervical spine is the upper two facet joints. There is no analogous structure in the thoracic spine. If, in addition to the spine pain, the individual is also experiencing leg or arm pain, then 95% of the time it is due to nerve root inflammation or compression. With this understanding, we can sort out and treat the various pain generators in the spine.

Epidural steroid injection is the most common spinal injection for relief of painful discs, or pain caused by nerve root inflammation. We insert a needle into the epidural space (the space between the two membranes that encase the spinal cord) and inject medication where the discs are pushing against nerve roots. This medication relieves the inflammation. These injections require fluoroscopic guidance for accurate needle placement. Usually we inject a mixture of local anesthetic and a depo-corticosteroid.

Epidural injections may be repeated two or three times in six months if there is an acceptable response. Since these are intra-spinal injections, serious complications can occur and have been reported. These include nerve damage, spinal injury, infection, bleeding, and spinal headache. Side effects from the steroids may include changes in blood sugar level, water retention, and hypertension. Fortunately, side effects and complications are rare and the procedure is well tolerated by most patients.

We use facet injections to diagnose and treat back pain caused by painful or inflamed facet joints. Facet joints are similar to other joints, like the knee joint, and can become painful for the same reasons: trauma, arthritis, and inflammation. Like any joint, a facet joint can be injected with medication. However, because facet joints are very small, injecting them requires special skill, training, and fluoroscopic guidance. Facet joint injections involve placing a very small gauge needle into the joint and injecting local anesthetic with a depo-corticosteroid to reduce inflammation and pain. We do sacroiliac joint injections the same way. These injections can be repeated in 6 to 8 weeks if there is a significant response.

Cryolesioning and Radiofrequency Lesioning

If facet injections provide excellent but only temporary relief, destroying the endings of the nerves transmitting pain can be considered. There are two techniques available: cryolesioning and radiofrequency lesioning.

Cryolesioning involves the use of very cold temperatures to freeze the nerve endings. We do this using a cryoprobe, a special instrument with a tip that reaches a temperature of −70 degrees Centigrade. We insert it through a catheter placed on the nerve endings of the painful facet joint. The intense cold is applied for 2 to 3 minutes to freeze the nerve endings. Transmission of pain will not occur until the nerve ending regenerates in about 4 weeks. In some patients the pain does not return for several months.

Radiofrequency lesioning is a similar technique, but instead of using intense cold, heat is applied to the nerve endings on the facet joints. This technique does cause more permanent destruction of the nerve endings, which often results in longer lasting pain relief than cryolesioning or facet injections. Typically, pain relief from radiofrequency lesioning lasts for several months in individuals suffering from severe facet joint pain.

Both cryolesioning and radiofrequency lesioning can be done in an outpatient setting, either in a surgical center or an office. Complications and side effects can occur but are rare. These include nerve damage, neuritis (nerve inflammation) or neuralgia (nerve pain), spinal injury, infection, bleeding, and spinal headache. Cryolesioning does not cause permanent injury to the nerve endings, so neuritis and neuralgia are unlikely to occur.

Intervertebral Disc Procedures

For disc pain that is unresponsive to conservative therapies, including epidural steroid injections, newer intervertebral disc technologies may be indicated. These technologies include intradiscal electrothermal annuloplasty (IDET) and percutaneous disc decompression. IDET involves heating the outer layer of the disc. Percutaneous disc decompression involves shrinking the center of the disc by heating or draining fluid.

To be successful with these treatments, we must know which discs are causing the pain. To find out, we do a discogram. Discography involves placing a needle into the suspected disc with the aid of fluoroscopy. Then we pressurize the discs using contrast dye while carefully measuring the pressure and observing whether the injection causes pain. Typically, a normal disc can be pressurized to 100 or 120 pounds per square inch without generating severe pain. Discs that generate pain at lower pressures are considered positive. Sometimes we do a CT scan immediately after the discogram for a more detailed picture of the discs.

Once a disc has been identified as the source of pain, we determine the specific abnormality. Only certain disc conditions can be successfully treated with these disc technologies. IDET is for the treatment of back pain due to small disc bulges or protrusions, with tears in the outer layer that are not severe enough to address through other types of spinal surgery. The therapy is not available for disc problems above the mid-chest level.

First, we place a needle into the painful disc, using fluoroscopy to guide us. Next, we insert a thermal probe through the needle into the disc and advance it over the bulge or tear. Using a radiofrequency generator attached to the thermal catheter, we apply heat to the outer layer of the disc, known as the annulus. Heating the annulus causes it to shrink, reducing the size of the bulge or tear and desensitizing the nerve endings to pain.

Complete healing of the disc takes up to 3 months. However, many notice pain relief within a few weeks after the procedure. IDET is a safe procedure and well tolerated by most patients. Serious complications can occur but are rare. These include infection, nerve damage, and spinal headache.

Percutaneous disc decompression is indicated for mild disc bulges, or protrusions, causing significant arm or leg pain. This technique is similar to IDET. We place an introducer needle into the painful disc, using fluoroscopic guidance. Next, we insert a decompression instrument into the disc through the needle. We remove 1 to 2 cubic centimeters of the disc's center, either mechanically or thermally. Doing so reduces the disc volume by 10–15%, enough to reduce nerve root compression and alleviate the arm or leg pain. Recovery is usually much faster than with IDET. Most patients feel improvement within a few days to a couple of weeks. The risks and complications are similar to those for IDET, but fortunately are rare.

Advanced Interventional Therapies

What if the pain is unremitting in spite of conservative therapy? What if surgery is not helpful or indicated? What if medications are ineffective or cause too many side effects? What options are left? In these situations, advanced interventional therapies may be the answer.

Advanced interventional therapy involves modulating the central nervous system, a process also called *neuromodulation*. This can be done in one of two ways.

The first technique involves using electrical stimulation to alter what the individual feels. We do this by delivering an electrical signal that prevents some of the pain from getting through the neural gates at the top of the spine. This technology is called *spinal cord stimulation*.

We place electrodes in the epidural space, the same area where epidural injections are given, using fluoroscopic guidance. We position the electrodes so that the patient feels a gentle massage or vibration in the same area where they usually feel the pain. The spinal cord stimulation impulses reach the brain faster than the pain signals from elsewhere in the body, so spinal cord stimulation fills some of the neural gates at the top of the spinal cord, thus blocking the pain with the more pleasant electrical stimulation.

Unfortunately, not all patients find the spinal cord stimulation sensation pleasant, so this treatment isn't right for everyone.

The advantage of this technology is that it is predictable and reversible. We run a 3- to 5-day outpatient trial in all potential candidates using percutaneous electrodes wired to a stimulator outside of the body. The trial must be successful before a complete system is surgically implanted. If necessary, the system can be completely removed.

Significant improvements in this technology have occurred over the past few years. There are now systems with rechargeable batteries that don't need to be replaced for several years. The best candidates for spinal cord stimulation are those who have some type of nerve injury or neuropathy, especially in the arms or legs.

Intrathecal pump therapy is the other form of neuromodulation. For this treatment we implant a small catheter into the spinal fluid sac and attach a tube from it to a pump reservoir placed under the skin of the waist. The spinal fluid sac connects to a canal that runs up the center of the spinal cord to the brain, so we can pump medication directly to the brain and spinal cord, where it is much more effective with potentially fewer side effects than when taken by mouth.

Intrathecal pump therapy is considered when a person requires high doses of oral or transdermal (patch-delivered) opioids for pain control and is experiencing inadequate relief with significant side effects. Successful trials using morphine or another potent opioid are required before installing the pump.

There is a battery-operated system that has the advantage of programmability, but requires replacement of the pump reservoir every few years. Another system uses a mechanical pump without a battery that doesn't need to be replaced, but is not programmable. These technologies are invasive and have significant risks and potential complications including nerve damage, spinal cord injury, infection, and spinal headache. Therefore, it is imperative that patients are well selected and are good candidates for these technologies to be successful.

In summary, fibromyalgia is a common chronic pain disorder that is usually described as widespread musculoskeletal aches and pains. Other symptoms may be associated with fibromyalgia including soft tissue swelling, muscle spasms, fatigue, sleep disturbances, restless legs syndrome, skin sensitivities, Raynaud's Syndrome, neurological symptoms, and impaired coordination. Many of the symptoms seen in fibromyalgia also occur in other common pain conditions including myofascial pain dysfunction syndrome and spinal pain. The cause of fibromyalgia still remains a mystery. Unfortunately, there are no specific diagnostics tests for fibromyalgia. Therefore, it is very important to rule out, and if necessary, treat these other conditions before diagnosing and treating fibromyalgia. Fortunately, there are now available new interventional pain treatment therapies, not only for relief of pain due to fibromyalgia, but also for many other common painful conditions.

Suggested Readings

Simons DG, Travell JG, Simons LS. *Myofascial Pain and Dysfunction: The Trigger Point Manual*. Philadelphia: Lippincott, 1999.

Starlanyl D, Copeland ME. *Fibromyalgia & Chronic Myofascial Pain—A Survival Manual*. Oakland: New Harbinger, 2001.

Waldman SD. *Atlas of Pain Management Injection Techniques*. Philadelphia: Saunders, 2000.

Waldman SD. *Atlas of Interventional Pain Management, 2nd Edition*. Philadelphia: Saunders, 2004.

CHAPTER 5

Pharmacology Management in Fibromyalgia

Randy Schad, RPh

Treating fibromyalgia requires a combination of pharmacological and nonpharmacological therapies. Many of the problems patients have are a consequence of chronic pain. Although eliminating all the pain isn't possible in most fibromyalgia patients, when it's even partially relieved, they get significant improvement in psychological distress, cognitive ability, sleep, and physical ability. Yet, they don't rely on pain medication exclusively.

A recent clinical review on fibromyalgia management supports the use of medications with exercise, cognitive therapy, patient education, and a multidisciplinary approach. The reviewers conducted a literature search of all human trials in the treatment of fibromyalgia. More than 500 articles were reviewed to provide evidence-based guidelines for the optimal treatment of fibromyalgia.[1]

Drug Therapy

Drug therapy plays a major role in the treatment of pain. Taking the medication(s) as directed and not missing doses is important. Some medications are taken on a regular schedule, whereas others are taken as needed, depending on the medication and the severity of the symptoms. A critical objective of drug therapy is to make patients see and believe that, through their actions, they can control their pain.

Three classes of medications can be used:

- Non-narcotic analgesics
- Narcotic analgesics
- Adjuvant medications—medications that are used to enhance the effect of analgesic prescribed medication (antidepressants and anticonvulsants)

The World Health Organization recommends a stepped approach to managing pain. During initial treatment, the lowest dose of a single agent is used. The dose is titrated to determine the effectiveness of the medication. If a single medication doesn't control the pain, an additional medication from another class is added. This method incorporates all three types of medications to maximize pain control. During each step, the patient is assessed to determine his or her response to the treatment. Sometimes medications are used together, even though a drug interaction or an adverse effect is possible. Your doctor should discuss these possible interactions or effects with you.

Now let's look at the medications used to treat fibromyalgia.

Non-Narcotic Analgesics

The non-narcotic analgesics include acetaminophen and a class of drugs called the nonsteroidal anti-inflammatory drugs, or NSAIDs.

Acetaminophen (Tylenol)

Acetaminophen (Tylenol) is the safest analgesic. It reduces fever and is an effective initial analgesic for mild pain. Studies show acetaminophen is as effective as ibuprofen (Motrin) in the short-term treatment of osteoarthritis in the knee, though it hasn't been studied in fibromyalgia as a single agent. For most patients, however, acetaminophen alone doesn't control the pain. Unlike NSAIDs, it doesn't reduce inflammation either. For added analgesic effect it is combined with narcotics or tramadol.

Mechanism of Action. We don't know exactly how acetaminophen works, but we think it affects the brain, It doesn't inhibit prostaglandin synthesis (the release of chemicals from cells that stimulate pain-sensing nerve fibers) like NSAIDs do.[2]

Adverse Effects. If taken at recommended doses, acetaminophen has no known stomach, kidney, or cardiovascular side effects. Hypersensitivity has been reported, and the reaction is usually a rash. Massive overdoses and long-term overuse have been reported to cause kidney damage.[3]

Dosing. The adult dose is 325–650 mg every 4 to 6 hours as needed. Don't conclude, after taking one or two doses, that acetaminophen is ineffective. You may need to take the appropriate dose for a week before benefiting. Doses greater than 4 grams (8 tablets of 500 mg each or 12 tablets of 325 mg each) per day, used for prolonged periods, have been associated with liver damage. In order to provide a margin of safety it would be prudent to keep the daily dose under 4 grams, or 4,000 mg, for someone who consumes a lot of over-the-counter medications. Acetaminophen is the active ingredient in more than 600 prescription and over-the-counter products. Therefore, consider the amount of acetaminophen you may be getting in any of these other medications when calculating your daily intake, so that you don't exceed the 4-gram limit.[4]

Precautions. Acetaminophen is not recommended for patients with a history of alcohol use (two or more drinks per day) or serious liver disease. It should be used cautiously in patients with renal (kidney) disease.[3]

Drug Interactions. No significant drug interactions have been identified, though there is (conflicting) information indicating that there may be increased risk of bleeding if warfarin (Coumadin) and acetaminophen are taken together.[3]

Tramadol

Tramadol (Ultram) is an analgesic that acts in the brain to alter pain perception. It has none of the kidney, gastrointestinal, and cardiovascular side effects associated with traditional and COX-2 nonsteroidal medications.

Clinical Trials. Tramadol has been studied for the treatment of fibromyalgia pain.[7,8,9] It was used either alone or in combination with acetaminophen (Ultracet), and was effective in three randomized clinical trials.

Mechanism of Action. Tramadol alters pain perception by binding weakly to the *mu* opioid receptors (nerves located in the brain and spinal cord that cause us to feel pain when stimulated) in the central nervous system and by inhibiting the re-uptake of serotonin and norepinephrine by nerve cells. It has no effect on prostaglandins and therefore has no anti-inflammatory properties.[2]

Adverse Effects. Adverse effects include nausea, vomiting, anxiety, increased sweating, rash, confusion, euphoria, and sleep disturbances. Other side effects include dizziness, drowsiness, fatigue, restlessness, and headache. Gastrointestinal problems include loss of appetite, constipation, and dry mouth.

Tramadol increases the risk of seizure and therefore should be used cautiously in patients:[3]

- With a history of seizures
- At increased risk of seizure (e.g., head trauma, alcohol withdrawal)
- Taking medication that decreases the seizure threshold, such as selective serotonin reuptake inhibitors (SSRIs), antidepressants, tricyclic antidepressants, neuroleptics (for mental illness), and monoamine oxidase (MAO) inhibitors (for depression).

Serotonin syndrome has been observed in patients taking tramadol with SSRIs. Symptoms include mental status changes, agitation, sweating, low blood pressure, nausea, shivering, tremor, diarrhea, lack of coordination, fever, muscle jerks, and hyperactive reflexes.

Dosing. Tramadol can be administered for pain in doses of 50 to 100 mg every 4 to 6 hours—not to exceed 400 mg per day. To decrease the incidence of side effects, patients troubled by nausea or vomiting should start with 25 to 50 mg and increase by 25 to 50 mg every 3 days, as tolerated, to 200 mg/day (50 mg, 4 times a day). For patients between the ages of 65 and 75 years, starting at one-half tablet and titrating the dose is recommended. For those over 75, the total dose should not exceed 300 mg per day. For those with severe liver or kidney disease, doses should be adjusted to 50 mg every 12 hours. You can take tramadol with or without food.[2]

Precautions. Abrupt discontinuation of tramadol may cause withdrawal symptoms, such as anxiety, sweating, hallucinations, nausea, tremors, or insomnia. Tapering the medication prevents these symptoms. Patients with a history of anaphylactoid reactions to codeine or other opioids may have an increased risk of such a reaction. Do not drive or operate machinery until you know how your body reacts to this drug.[2]

Drug Interactions. Drug interactions are possible. Ask your doctor or pharmacist before using any other medicines along with tramadol. This includes over-the-counter medications and herbal products.[2]

Availability. Tramadol is available as a generic medication. Each tablet contains 50 mg of tramadol. When combined with acetaminophen, only the trade name product, Ultracet, is available. This combination product contains 37.5 mg of tramadol and 325 mg of acetaminophen. It is now available as a long-acting formulation.

Nonsteroidal Anti-inflammatory Drugs (NSAIDs)

NSAIDs are commonly used in the treatment of fibromyalgia, but they haven't been proved effective when used alone.[1] However, they may be useful adjuncts for analgesia when combined with tricyclic antidepressants. In addition, fibromyalgia patients may have other painful conditions. NSAIDs are effective against acute and chronic pain, inflammatory musculoskeletal conditions, headache, and fever.

Because of potential severe long-term side effects, NSAIDs should be used for the shortest time possible.

There are more than 20 NSAIDs, including aspirin and the controversial COX-2 selective NSAIDs. In terms of pain relief, one NSAID has no advantage over another. Patients who don't respond to one NSAID may respond to a medication in another class. Unless side effects warrant changing, patients should be started on at least a 2-week trial of an NSAID before switching to another. Tolerance and physical dependence do not develop with NSAIDs.

Mechanism of Action. NSAIDs inhibit cyclooxygenase (COX), an enzyme that catalyzes a step in the synthesis of prostaglandins, which cause inflammation. Two forms of COX have been identified, COX-1 and COX-2. COX-1 is normally present in the stomach's inner lining and is involved in the production of prostaglandins that produce a protective barrier of mucus and bicarbonate. COX-1 plays a role in kidney function and is also present in the kidneys and blood platelets (cells that aid in clotting). COX-2 is present in the kidneys, the central nervous system (brain and spinal cord), and inflamed tissues. It is responsible for pain regulation and inflammation. The ideal NSAID would inhibit only COX-2 and exert no effect on COX-1.[2]

Adverse Effects. Adverse effects of these medications are related to their mechanism of action, inhibition of prostaglandin synthesis. In addition, there are medical conditions that can increase the risk for experiencing side effects.

The most common adverse effects are gastrointestinal (GI) problems, including dyspepsia, abdominal pain, and nausea. GI ulcers and bleeding are common and can be very serious, leading to hospitalization and death. They often occur without warning symptoms in patients treated with NSAIDs. All members of the NSAID family of drugs (including COX-2s) can cause GI toxicity. The risk of GI toxicity from these drugs increases with increasing doses and the length of treatment.

If the following symptoms develop while taking NSAIDs, stop taking them and contact a physician immediately:

- Severe abdominal pain
- Cramping or burning
- Severe and continuing nausea
- Heartburn or bloating
- Black, tarry, or bloody stools
- Vomiting blood or material that looks like coffee grounds

Occasionally patients also develop dizziness, confusion, or headache.[3]

Precautions. Blood counts, renal function, and liver enzymes should be checked periodically. There is little evidence that NSAIDs protect against heart attack or stroke. NSAIDs may be used with low-dose aspirin, but doing so may increase the risk of gastric bleeding or ulcers. If NSAIDs cause stomach distress, taking a proton pump inhibitor (stomach acid inhibitor) such as lansoprazole (Prevacid) or omeprazole (Prilosec) will prevent ulcers. Misoprostol (Cytotec) may also be prescribed to reduce the risk of stomach ulcers and promote the healing of existing ones. This medication is expensive, and its side effects of bloating and diarrhea may limit its use. To minimize the risk of NSAID-related stomach problems, avoid drinking alcohol and take medications with food and a full glass of water. Many over-the-counter cold and pain medications include the NSAID ibuprofen, so combining these medications with prescription NSAIDs may increase the chance of experiencing an adverse effect.[3]

Drug Interactions. Ask your doctor or pharmacist before using any other medications with NSAIDs. This includes over-the-counter medications and herbal products. NSAIDs decrease the efficacy of diuretics, beta blockers, and ace inhibitors (blood pressure medications), thereby raising blood pressure. Because they increase the chance of bleeding (an inadequate clotting response to little leaks in the bloodstream), NSAIDs should be used cautiously in patients taking medications that affect platelets (clotting components in the blood)—medications like aspirin and clopidegel (Plavix), and blood thinners like warfarin (Coumadin). Other drugs, such as corticosteroids, that increase the risk of stomach ulcers should also be used cautiously.[3]

Narcotic Analgesics

The best-known class of medications to treat pain is the narcotic analgesics. There are two types of narcotics, the opioids and the opiates. Opioids are synthetic narcotics that resemble opiates in action but aren't derived from opium. Opiates *are* prepared or derived from opium.

There have been no randomized, controlled trials of narcotic analgesics in patients with fibromyalgia.[1] These drugs should be prescribed only if (1) all medicinal and nonmedicinal therapies produce inadequate pain relief and (2) the patient's quality of life is affected by the pain. A physician who specializes in pain medicine should be consulted.

Narcotic analgesics are accepted as highly effective in managing acute pain and cancer-related pain. They are gradually gaining acceptance for use against chronic nonmalignant pain. The American Pain Society and the American Academy of Pain Medicine state that using narcotics to manage chronic nonmalignant pain is appropriate when other available strategies have produced inadequate relief. However, many physicians, nurses, and pharmacists fear addiction and other drug-related behaviors. This is also a common fear of many patients and family members.

Mechanism of Action. All narcotics have an affinity for opioid receptors in the brain, spinal cord, and gastrointestinal tract. By binding to these receptors, they block transmission of noxious stimuli to the brain. The two main receptors responsible for analgesia (i.e., pain killing) are the *mu* opioid receptors (found in the brain, spinal cord, and smooth muscles throughout the body) and the *kappa* opioid receptors. They are also involved in adverse effects like sedation, constipation, respiratory depression, and intoxication. Narcotics have no effect on prostaglandin and therefore no anti-inflammatory properties. Unlike the NSAIDs, they don't cause GI bleeding and have no renal or cardiovascular effects.[3]

Adverse Effects. All narcotics have adverse effects like somnolence (needing too much sleep), confusion, euphoria, constipation, drowsiness, nausea, vomiting, respiratory depression (shallow breathing), hypotension (low blood pressure), itching, and urinary retention.

Yet the body quickly adapts, developing a tolerance to the drug that reduces some of these effects. Tolerance to sedation, respiratory depression, and nausea and vomiting develop within a few days or weeks, although patients with severe nausea may need an antiemetic (antinausea) to control it. Sedation usually occurs only at the beginning of therapy or when the dosage is increased. Tolerance to constipation never develops, so stool softeners or laxatives are needed.[3]

Many people confuse the terms *addiction, physical dependence,* and *tolerance.* Actually, each phenomenon has different pharmacological effects on the body. To use narcotics against chronic pain properly and effectively, you need to understand the difference.

> *Addiction* is characterized by one or more of the following behaviors: lack of control regarding drug use, compulsive use, continued use despite harm, and craving.

> *Physical dependence* means that the body becomes accustomed to the medication. Abrupt cessation, rapid dose reduction, decreasing blood level of the medication, and/or administration of an antagonist (a medication that reverses the effect of a previously administered medication) can cause patients to experience withdrawal symptoms such as diarrhea, sweating, nausea, vomiting, nasal congestion, seizures, and depression.

> *Tolerance* is the reduction in a medication's effects over time. Tolerance to analgesia of a narcotic is uncommon once long-term pain relief has been achieved. Some tolerance is desirable (i.e. when the sedative, nausea, and mental clouding side effects of narcotics subside during dose titration).

The American Pain Society has defined addiction, physical dependence, and tolerance. Please refer to its web site for the most up-to-date definitions (http://www.ampainsoc.org/advocacy/opioids2.htm).

Availability. Additional pain relief can be gained by combining narcotic medications with acetaminophen or an NSAID like aspirin. If one narcotic provides inadequate pain relief or causes troublesome side effects, starting a trial of a second narcotic may prove beneficial.

Precautions. Whenever you start taking a narcotic or have your dosage increased, avoid driving or operating machinery until you develop tolerance to any side effects. Abrupt discontinuation of narcotics causes withdrawal symptoms. Don't split, crush, or chew extended release tablets and capsules. If a prolonged daily narcotic regimen is discontinued for a period of time, it may be dangerous to immediately resume the dosage that existed prior to the stoppage.[3]

Drug Interactions. Because narcotics depress activity in the brain and spinal cord, increased depressant effects occur if narcotics are taken with other medications that depress the central nervous system, such as antihistamines (allergy medications), tranquilizers, sleeping medications, tricyclic antidepressants, muscle relaxants, other narcotic pain medications, and alcohol. Ask your doctor or pharmacist before using any other medication with a narcotic. This includes over-the-counter medications and herbal medications.[3]

Medication Contracts. Physicians may have you sign a "Medication Management Agreement," which is a contract between the physician and you. In it you agree to always use the same pharmacy, to use only one physician to prescribe the narcotics, and to call for refills only during regular business hours. Most physicians require patients be seen by a psychologist to help you develop behavioral pain management strategies. Involvement in the behavioral pain management aspect of the program is important in preventing the development of tolerance to the analgesic effects of the narcotic medications.

Adjuvant Therapies

Adjuvant therapies are drugs that augment the effects of analgesics. They include antidepressants and anticonvulsants.

Antidepressants

Antidepressants inhibit the reuptake of neurotransmitters (serotonin, norepinephrine, and dopamine) that cause the level of neurotransmitters to increase. They are thought to have an actual analgesic effect, not just a psychological effect. The three types of antidepressant drugs are:

- Tricyclic antidepressants
- Selective serotonin reuptake inhibitors
- Serotonin and norepinephrine reuptake inhibitors

Tricyclic Antidepressants. Tricyclic antidepressants are useful and effective in treating chronic pain syndromes. Amitriptyline (Elavil) and cyclobenzaprine (Flexeril) have been shown to be very efficacious in treating fibromyalgia.[8-14] Randomized, controlled trials show that 10 to 50 mg of amitriptyline at bedtime are effective. Cyclobenzaprine is marketed as a muscle relaxant, but structurally it is a tricyclic. In randomized, controlled trials lasting 6 to 12 weeks, patients given 10 to 40 mg per day found it effective.

MECHANISM OF ACTION. Researchers believe that the tricyclic antidepressants have an analgesic effect by inhibiting the reuptake of norepinephrine and serotonin, which are chemicals that transmit electrical currents from one nerve cell to another in parts of the brain and spinal cord.[3]

ADVERSE EFFECTS. Adverse effects of the tricyclic antidepressants include dry mouth, decreased tear flow, constipation, weight gain, urinary retention, blurred vision, skin rashes, jaundice, sexual dysfunction, and persistent daytime somnolence. Central nervous system effects may impede balance, gait, and attention levels. These drugs may worsen narrow-angle glaucoma. Other potentially dangerous adverse effects include arrhythmias and abnormalities that prevent the muscle cells of the heart from contracting in an efficient, synchronized pattern. Tricyclics are associated with a risk of seizure and should be used cautiously in patients with a history of seizures, in those at increased risk for seizure, and in those taking other drugs that decrease the seizure threshold. (See also the adverse effects of tramadol above and of SSRIs below.)[3]

DOSING. Amitriptyline is taken in doses of 25 to 50 mg at bedtime. Some recommend taking it 2 to 3 hours before bedtime, so that you're drowsy at bedtime. Patients may adjust the timing of doses to minimize side effects and maximize benefit. Expect to wait 1 to 3 weeks for maximum sleep modification and analgesic effect. If increased doses are needed, titrations can be given at 10-mg increments. Some patients may need to decrease the dose to 10 mg if sedation or other side effects are too severe. If an even smaller dose is needed, you can split a 10-mg tablet in half with a tablet cutter. If the side effects persist, your doctor might switch you to another tricyclic antidepressant.

Doses recommended for fibromyalgia are much smaller than the doses used to treat depression. For patients who need to be slowly titrated on the medication, doxepin (10 mg/ml) is available as a liquid. Cyclobenzaprine in doses of 10 to 30 mg should also be taken at bedtime, though the dose and time can be reduced by the patient. Most patients develop a tolerance to the daytime sedation.

PRECAUTIONS. Tricyclics may impair mental and/or physical abilities, so use caution when performing hazardous tasks or operating machinery. Abrupt discontinuation may cause gastrointestinal distress, restlessness, or sleep disturbances characterized by vivid and colorful dreams. You can prevent these problems by tapering the dosage over 5 to 10 days. These agents should be used with extreme caution in patients 65 and older, because they increase the potential for confusion, disorientation, and hallucinations. Nearly all antidepressant medications are eliminated through the liver, so they should be used with caution in patients with liver problems.[3]

DRUG INTERACTIONS. Tricyclics depress activity in the brain and spinal cord, so increased depressant effects occur if they are taken with other medications that depress the central nervous system, such as antihistamines, tranquilizers, sleep medications, narcotics, muscle relaxants, and alcohol. To avoid serious adverse effects, don't take tricyclics with MAO inhibitors such as selegiline (Eldepryl), phenelzine (Nardil), and tranylcypromine (Parnate).

The combined use of tricyclic antidepressants and SSRIs like Zoloft, Paxil, and Prozac may inhibit the natural breakdown of the tricyclic, leading to increased levels of it, increased side effects, and serotonin syndrome. (See the drug interactions of tramadol above and SSRIs below.)

Ask your doctor or pharmacist before using any other medicine along with the SSRIs or tricyclic antidepressants. This includes over-the-counter medications and herbal products.

Selective Serotonin Reuptake Inhibitors (SSRIs)/Serotonin Norepinephrine Reuptake Inhibitors (SNRIs) There is some evidence to indicate that other antidepressant medications may be helpful in treating fibromyalgia.[15-18] These include the selective serotonin reuptake inhibitors (SSRIs), like Prozac and Zoloft. Although they appear useful, the SSRIs and other antidepressants haven't been studied as extensively as amitriptyline (Elavil) and cyclobenzaprine (Flexeril), so further study is needed.

Another group of antidepressants are the serotonin and norepinephrine reuptake inhibitors (SNRIs). They selectively block the reabsorption of both serotonin and norepinephrine so they are sometimes known as dual reuptake inhibitors. Venlafaxine (Effexor), duloxetine (Cymbalta), and milnacipran (Ixel) belong to this group.

- Milnacipran (Ixel) is not yet available in the United States. However, it was shown to be more effective than placebo in improving pain scores in patients who participated in one clinical trial that lasted 12 weeks.[19] Adverse effects that were experienced by patients leading to discontinuing therapy included headache, GI complaints, orthostatic dizziness, elevated blood pressure, depression, lethargy, sweating, and hot flashes.
- Two small studies found venlafaxine (Effexor) useful. The first showed that 6 out of 11 depressed patients who completed 8 weeks of therapy experienced at least a 50% reduction in fibromyalgia symptoms.[20] These included significantly improved pain, less fatigue, better sleep, less morning stiffness, less depression and anxiety, and better patient global assessment scores. Patients received doses ranging from 37.5 mg to 300 mg per day. The most frequent side effects were insomnia, headache, constipation, fatigue, nausea, and dry mouth. The second study found similar results.[21] Fifteen

patients completed a 12-week trial on a fixed dose of 75 mg per day. There were significant improvements in the mean intensity of pain (average daily pain ratings based on a 0–10 scale) and in the disability caused by fibromyalgia.

- Over 12 weeks, duloxetine (Cymbalta), a dual serotonin and norepinephrine reuptake inhibitor, was found to work better than a placebo in 207 patients with fibromyalgia.[22] Duloxetine improved fibromyalgia symptoms and pain severity regardless of the baseline level of depression. The patients were titrated upward over 2 weeks, starting with 20 mg every day for 5 days, then 20 mg twice daily for 3 days, then 40 mg twice daily for 3 days, then 40 mg twice daily for two days, and finally 60 mg twice daily for the rest of the study. They reported problems with insomnia, dry mouth, and constipation more frequently than patients who took a placebo.

  In a second randomized double-blind placebo-controlled study, duloxetine was found to be better than placebo in 354 patients with fibromyalgia.[23] Compared to patients who took placebos, patients treated with either 60 mg once a day or 60 mg twice a day of duloxetine for 12 weeks had significantly greater improvement in pain scores and other measured outcomes. Patients in the duloxetine groups reported nausea, diarrhea, dry mouth, somnolence, feeling jittery, sweating, nervousness, constipation, decreased appetite, and anorexia significantly more frequently than did the placebo-treated patients.

DRUG INTERACTIONS. SSRIs may cause drug interactions because they inhibit enzyme systems in the liver that break down other medications. These medications then accumulate faster than the body can dispose of them. This can lead to higher drug concentrations and potentially increased pharmacological effects and increased adverse side effects. SSRI drug interactions have been reported with alprazolam (Xanax), the tricyclic antidepressants, warfarin (Coumadin), MAO inhibitors, clozapine (Clozaril), phenytoin (Dilantin), carbamazepine (Tegretol), and theophylline.

Again, ask your doctor or pharmacist before using any other medicine along with the SSRIs or tricyclic antidepressants. This includes over-the-counter medications and herbal products.[3]

Anticonvulsants

Anticonvulsants are used to treat epilepsy. They are also useful against neuropathic pain. Gabapentin (Neurontin) is the best-studied and best-tolerated anticonvulsant for the neuropathic pain associated with diabetic neuropathy, postherpetic neuralgia, mixed neuropathic pain syndromes, phantom limb pain, Guillain-Barre syndrome, and the acute and chronic pain from spinal cord injuries.

Gabapentin is currently undergoing randomized control trials in treating fibromyalgia. However, pregabalin (Lyrica), related to gabapentin, has been found effective in treating fibromyalgia in a randomized, double-blind placebo-controlled trial.[24] The 8-week study compared various doses of pregabalin in 529 patients. Compared with those who took the placebo, those who took up to 450 mg per day reported reduced average severity of pain. More of them also reported more than 50% improvement in pain. This study also found improvement in sleep, fatigue, and health-related quality of life. Seventy-eight percent of the patients completed the trial and entered a follow-on safety trial. The most common adverse effects were dizziness and somnolence.

Adverse Effects. The most common side effects are somnolence, fatigue, dizziness, tremor, double vision, blurred vision, amnesia, involuntary eye movements, and ataxia. These effects frequently resolve within a few weeks of treatment. Other adverse effects include weight gain, lower extremity swelling, nausea, constipation, depression, dry mouth, and upset stomach.[3]

Dosing. The starting dose of gabapentin is usually 100 to 300 mg taken at bedtime. The dosage then is increased gradually every 3 days over 4 to 8 weeks to a maximum of 2,400 to 3,600 mg per day in three divided doses. Dosages should be titrated upward until adverse effects occur, then reduced to the dosage at which they no longer occur.[3]

Precautions. Use cautiously in patients 65 and over, and patients with impaired kidney function.

Drug Interactions. There are no significant drug interactions with gabapentin. Added sedation may occur when using it with other medications that depress the central nervous system. Antacids given concurrently with gabapentin reduce its absorption by 20%. If antacids are taken, gabapentin should be taken 2 hours later.[3]

Potential Herbal and Prescription Medication Interaction

Predicting drug interactions with herbal products is problematic for two reasons. First, herbal products aren't regulated by the Food and Drug Administration. Second, there is no quality control in the manufacturing process, so every ingredient in the herbal products isn't known and listed on the label, and the relative amounts of the substances can vary widely from batch to batch. So, always check with your pharmacist or physician before using prescription and herbal medications together.

Conclusion

Managing fibromyalgia pain is often frustrating for both the patient and the health care provider. Many different medications have been used to treat the pain. Published studies have shown them effective in controlling it, but the trials have been short ones, and improvement does not occur in every patient. For best results, pain medication should be used with nonmedicinal treatments, such as physical therapy, psychological support, and educational programs.

References

1. Goldenberg DL, Burckhardt A, Crofford L. Management of fibromyalgia syndrome. *JAMA.* 2004;292:2388-2395.
2. Hardman JG, Limbird LE, Gilman AG. *Goodman & Gilman's The Pharmacological Basis of Therapeutics.* 11th ed. New York: McGraw Hill; 2006:693.

3. Micromedex, Thomson Healthcare, Inc. Full text drug information databases. Available at: http://www.library.ucsf.edu/db/record.html? idrecord=82. Accessed <DATE>.

4. *Physicians Desk Reference.* Montvale NJ: Thomson; 2006:1843-1844.

5. Biasi G, Manaca S, Manganelli S. Tramadol in the treatment of fibromyalgia syndrome: a controlled clinical trial versus placebo. *Int J Clin Pharmacol Res.* 1998;18:13-19.

6. Russell J, Kamin M, Bennett RM. Efficacy of tramadol in treatment of pain in fibromyalgia. *J Clin Rheumatol.* 2000;6:250-257.

7. Bennett RM, Kamin M, Karin R. Tramadol and acetaminophen combination tablets in the treatment of fibromyalgia pain. *Am J Med.* 2003;114:537-545.

8. Carette S, McCain GA, Bell DA. Evaluation of amitriptyline in primary fibrositis. *Arthritis Rheum.* 1986;29:655-659.

9. Goldenberg DL, Felson DT, Dinerman HA. Randomized, controlled trial of amitriptyline and naproxen in the treatment of patients with fibromyalgia. *Arthritis Rheum.* 1986;29:1371-1377.

10. Carette S, Bell MJ, Reynolds WJ. Comparison of amitriptyline, cyclobenzaprine, and placebo in the treatment of fibromyalgia: a randomized, double-blind clinical trial. *Arthritis Rheum.* 1994;37:32-40.

11. Bennett RM, Gatter RA, Campbell SM. A comparison of cyclobenzaprine and placebo in the management of fibrositis. *Arthritis Rheum.* 1988;31:1535-1542.

12. Tofferi JK, Jackson JL, O'Malley PG. Treatment of fibromyalgia with cyclobenzaprine: a meta-analysis. *Arthritis Rheum.* 2004;51:9-13.

13. Arnold LM, Keck PE. Antidepressant treatment of fibromyalgia: a meta-analysis and review. *Psychosomatics.* 2000;41:104-113.

14. O'Malley PG, Balden E, Tomkins G. Treatment of fibromyalgia with antidepressants. *J Gen Intern Med.* 2000;15:659-666.

15. Wolfe F, Cathery MA, Hawley DJA. Double-blind placebo controlled trial of fluoxetine in fibromyalgia. *Scand J Rheumatol.* 1994;23:255-259.

16. Arnold LM, Hess EV, Hudson JL. Randomized, placebo-controlled, double-blind, flexible-dose study of fluoxetine in the treatment of women with fibromyalgia. *Am J Med.* 2002;112:191-197.

17. Goldenberg D, Mayskiy M, Mossey CJ. Randomized double-blind cross over trial of fluoxetine and amitriptyline in the treatment of fibromyalgia. *Arthritis Rheum.* 1996;39:1852-1859.

18. Celiker R, Cagavi Z. Comparison of amitriptyline and sertraline in the treatment of fibromyalgia syndrome [abstract]. *Arthritis Rheum.* 2000;43:s332.

19. Gendreau RM, Mease PJ, Rao SR. Minacipran: a potential new treatment of fibromyalgia [abstract]. *Arthritis Rheum.* 2003;48:s616.
20. Dwight MM, Arnold LM, O'Brien H. An open clinical trial of venlafaxine treatment of fibromyalgia. *Psychosomatics.* 1998;39:14-17.
21. Sayar K, Aksu G, Ak L. Venlafaxine treatment of fibromyalgia. *Ann Pharmacother.* 2003;37:1561-1565.
22. Arnold LM, Lu Y, Crofford LJ. A double-blind multicenter trial comparing duloxetine to placebo in the treatment of fibromyalgia with or without major depressive disorder. *Arthritis Rheum.* 2004;50:2974-2984.
23. Arnold LM, Rosen A, Pritchett Y. A randomized, double-blind, placebo-controlled trial of duloxetine in the treatment of women with fibromyalgia with or without major depressive disorder. *Pain.* 2005;119:5-15.
24. Crofford LJ, Rowbotham MC, Mease PJ. Pregabalin for the treatment of fibromyalgia sydrome: results of a randomized, double-blind, placebo-controlled trial. *Arthritis Rheum.* 2005;52:1264-1273.

CHAPTER 6

Growing Up, Living with, and Managing Fibromyalgia

Jerry Sauve

Jerry has graduated high school and is currently attending college as a full time student. He is pursuing a major in education, and would like to eventually teach high school English. Jerry continues to enjoy a full life without the stress and fatigue of fibromyalgia.

— •◆• —

My name is Jerry Sauve. I am 18 years old and pass my days either working part-time at the Detroit Zoo or spending time with my girl-friend and her family. I also try to get out at least once or twice a week to play two grueling hours of hockey with friends. I'm an all-around athletic guy, known in most of my circles for being the comedian . . . or the kid who won $1,000 and a brand new Corvette. But that's another story. (All right, all right, I only won the car for a week, but at least I've got your attention.)

In a little more than a month I start my freshman year of college. I plan to teach at the high school where I spent my freshman and sophomore years barely keeping my head above water.

Oh yeah, there's one other thing—I have fibromyalgia.

Somehow, though, life is very normal. I have a job, I have a girlfriend, and I go to sleep every night and wake up every morning, grumbling as one might expect. I go out with my friends and play a little hockey whenever we can all fit it into our schedules—schedules busy at this time in our lives when we find ourselves suddenly overwhelmed with responsibilities we never would've thought ourselves (or each other) capable of.

Yes, my life is what you'd expect for any 18 year old you might know, and yet, here I am in the middle of this book about fibromyalgia, and you're wondering why.

It started when I was about 8 years old, and it lasted (at full force) until about two years ago. It stopped rather suddenly. (Or, at least I feel close enough to "normal" that I would hardly know the difference.)

From birth to around age 8, I was a reasonably healthy child. You could probably say I was a bit sensitive, even as young children go. I started second grade in a new school, a much smaller school, when I first started getting sick. At first, it just seemed like I was a natural magnet for whatever flu was going around. I constantly had the flu, a cold, an ear infection, a sinus infection, stomach problems, or I just didn't feel good for one reason or another. All the same stuff other kids have, but with little time in between. Nonetheless, I still did well in school.

During third grade, my school absences really started to concern my parents. I was home sick a lot. So what's a lot, you ask? At that time I missed school for a week at the most, usually three to four days once or twice a month. Then in fourth grade I think it escalated to five days at a time, but not as often, just once a month. Again, it was always the flu or a cold, with stomach pain, muscle aches, joint pain, and exhaustion, though I had fewer ear infections and sinus infections than before.

Sound familiar?

After fourth grade, my absences became enough of a problem that my parents considered home-schooling me. It seemed that I was much better in the afternoon than in the morning. Home-schooling would let me sleep an extra hour or two without missing classroom instruction and having to make up the homework. (Make-up work piled up during a five-day absence.) Needless to say, we thought it made sense to give home-schooling a shot. Can't be absent when I'm home, right? Plus, it's no secret that the worst place for your kid to be when flus and colds are going around is public school, so being at home seemed like a smart move across the board.

By the end of home-schooling for the fifth grade, having had almost nothing educational happen, my parents decided I should go back to public school. We thought that maybe a year off had built up my immune system and had made me stronger. I'd recently learned how to ride a bike and had been out riding daily. This combination of exercise, fresh air, and plenty of sleep was a big step in the right direction.

I probably was the strongest I'd been in my life. Though I was keenly aware of how much school I had missed, I still didn't really consider myself sick—just unlucky. I'd gotten so used to my condition that I really hadn't thought much about all the time in doctors' offices and hospitals, except that it was no fun and that I was glad to be done with it. I felt pretty confident that I was.

I was excited about going back to public school, especially middle school. Although I was starting late in November, the late start worked out well for me. Plus, I share my first name with Jerry Springer, and this was at the height of his show's popularity. Since the pre-teen demographic gravitates toward all things absurd and in poor taste, for the first several months I had my entire grade chanting my name in the hallways like Springer's audience chants "Jer-ry!" on the show.

You can imagine my delight. Unfortunately, I bet it wasn't a month before I started getting sick again, missing several days or a week at a time. Before long, a week at a time became two weeks, two weeks became three, and by seventh grade, weeks became months. Yes, months.

I struggled. I was torn; physically and mentally, I was overwhelmed. Although I was still relatively healthy, I struggled under the load of excessive homework. Now I had three to five hours a night on top of being sick.

I fell so far behind that by the time I started something, the rest of the class was finishing it. Whether I went to school hardly mattered, because it was virtually impossible for me to catch up, much less participate. In addition to this pressure, other factors began to weigh in.

First, I couldn't just be one of "them" anymore. If it's been a while since your school days, I remind you how important it is to *not* be different. Even if you don't fit in, you can get by, so long as you don't stand out. And nothing makes you stand out more than being gone for a month or more at a time—while everyone thinks you died or are in the hospital—and then returning out of the blue.

Fortunately, when I was actually at school, I was both "the sick kid" and "the really funny kid." I knew that if I could ever stop being sick, I could be "the really funny kid who used to be sick all of the time," which was a definite and glorious upgrade, if indeed it was in reach.

Unfortunately, it simply wasn't. By eighth grade, I'd missed almost all but the first two or three months and the final two weeks of the year. There were kids who had actually forgotten about me, that I had to reintroduce myself to. These were kids I'd gone to school with for two years already! Ouch indeed.

The usual response when I was remembered, was "Oh man, I heard you'd died." I am serious. And after awhile, I would hardly blink. It became the expected, the assumed. Worse yet was that I didn't have a label for what was wrong with me and why I was never there. I didn't have a name for the disease I struggled against, something that people could understand. I know that a lot of people, young and old, probably didn't even believe I was sick.

Between the hours of homework I could never keep up with and being sick, I spent all my time indoors alone, wondering why I was sick all the time and whether I'd ever have a normal life. I went out of my way to avoid spending time with other people, because I'd closed myself off to the rest of the world in frustration, depression, and self-loathing. Then there were all the doctors' appointments, spending three hours in waiting rooms. Eventually I gave up on Western medicine altogether, though I appreciate the few doctors who legitimately tried and cared and were frustrated in their efforts to discover what direction to take treatment, in what form, against what condition, and so on.

Starting my sophomore year, I was determined not to miss school, no matter how hard it was, no matter how sick I was. But that goal just wasn't realistic. I still couldn't fall asleep at night and would only *begin* getting drowsy by morning. Therefore, it was nearly impossible for me to stay awake until the end of the day, much less pay attention and retain anything. The muscle aches and the joint pain were worst in the morning, and lack of sleep made them worse. I had stomach problems as well. After almost every meal I was nauseous, my stomach in knots. And I was losing weight.

Since then, I found that part of my stomach problem was due to an allergy to gluten (which is found in all wheat, grains, and oats). By eliminating gluten from my diet my stomach began to behave itself, but the pain and sleep problems persisted.

So, there I was starting my sophomore year, trying to get through a full week of school on little or no sleep, exhausted, with muscle aches and joint pain thrown in to take care of any dull moments. This was simply not a realistic routine for me, and again I found myself way over my head and well past my limit. I finally decided I'd had enough.

I had a long talk with my mother in which I pleaded my case, and she agreed to take me out of school. I needed to be able to sleep whenever I could and to get as much rest as I needed. I also needed to cut down on the incredible amount of stress and pressure of homework and grades. I needed to take care of myself, get control of my life, and take it from there. I was too sick too often, and I had zero quality of life. I'd come home from school and collapse, finally catching up on my sleep, only to wake up after dark and missing any opportunity for social interaction, but with an intimidating pile of homework to get through and only hours before I'd be back at school. Oh yeah, and eat something at some point.

So, I dropped out of school and proceeded to wait all night to be able to fall asleep around 9 or 10 in the morning, and then sleep all day. This is not as much fun as it sounds. Believe me, when your parent(s) have to get up for work in the morning, you are severely limited in what you can do on a schedule that has you awake all night and asleep all day.

What? Do you think you're gonna go outside and play basketball? In the dark? Going to go take a walk at four in the morning? So the cops can wake your parents when they bring you home? Going to watch television all night and just have a little party all by yourself? Do you have any idea how *bad* television gets after midnight? Do you have any idea the violent fits I'm thrown into at the mere hint of an infomercial?

But things soon got better. A great weight was lifted from my shoulders (not to mention my body) when I was freed of all the stress of the homework, of the bad grades, of always being behind, and of never doing anything good enough for anyone. With all that gone, I started sleeping.

Before that, I would get so tired of being tired I would just slip into unconsciousness and emerge from it 10 hours later like a mummy. There's a difference between that and actually "getting some sleep."

For the first time, I actually started to sleep well. Every day I fell asleep earlier. Before this, to reset my internal clock for the school week, I'd stay up Saturday night to try to fall asleep on Sunday night. Not that I'd wake rested or functional Monday morning, because this practice screwed me up for about four days afterward, but it was the only way I thought I could get back on a normal sleeping schedule.

Needless to say, that just didn't work. But now, I was falling asleep 10–15 minutes earlier every night, and soon I was falling asleep earlier than I ever had! At eight o'clock in the evening I was going to bed; at six o'clock in the morning I was waking up feeling like a million bucks. And the better sleep I got, the more manageable the pain was in my muscles and joints. The more manageable the pain got, the more I was up to doing during the day, and the better I felt inside and out. In other words, sleeping well made all the difference in the world. And that was just the beginning.

The more I took care of myself and learned to listen to my body (you have my word that "listening to your body" is more than an obnoxious, beaten-to-death medical cliché), the better things got. Suddenly, I wasn't feeling bad at all. And I could start taking steps towards getting my life back together.

I started home-schooling again, now old enough and close enough to the finish line that I could motivate myself to teach myself, through a wonderful program called the American School.

Amazingly, just a year later, here I am: 18 years old, with a girl-friend of two years, attending college, playing hockey with my friends, going to bed every night and waking up every morning, holding down a good job, and genuinely enjoying life. Life is so good that sometimes, I wonder if fibromyalgia's still in my system anymore. And then, every once in a while, I'll wake up with a very clear reminder that it is. And at certain points of the day, I still feel it, some days worse than others, depending on where I've been and what I've done; but this is *nothing* compared to being unable to function and enjoy life. After all, everyone has limitations.

So what's the secret? What's my advice for someone my age or younger who's struggling with school, with life, or in any way with fibromyalgia?

Look, there is no secret. It's common sense:

- First, know that whatever you have to do, you're going to survive.
- Take care of *yourself* first, and let the rest fall into place. If you can't handle the life that you're trying to live, figure out what changes you need to make and make them. Think outside the box.
- If you have trouble sleeping like I did, discuss it with your parents, your physician, and anyone else who could help you.
- Finally, consider home-schooling if you're ready for it.

Home-schooling is different. You get a diploma, and it's certified by educators who run the school and recognized by most institutions of higher education. It's just a different way for people who want another way. Or need one.

Home-schooling isn't the answer for every young person with fibromyalgia. Yet everyone has parts of their daily life that fibromyalgia makes sensationally difficult, and the best advice I can give is to explore your options. Never forget that you *have* options. They are endless. Talk with your doctor, talk with your family.

You go to a doctor for help, but sometimes there's not a lot they can do, especially for something like fibromyalgia. Even when they can help you, you need to look for other things that you can do to help yourself. Everyone is different, every body is different, but some things are universally easy, and listening to your body is one of them.

On that note, figure out when it's OK to push yourself and when it's not. Part of listening to your body is learning your limits. One trick to this is getting into good routines. Try to maintain as tight a sleep pattern as you can. Try to set times where you will not go to bed any later than this, and you will not wake up any later than that, and for your sake, keep them reasonable—at least eight hours per day.

I would also like to bring up a common grievance among fibromyalgia sufferers: that we are not always taken seriously, because we don't look as sick as we feel—if we look sick at all. Because of that some people don't believe that we are suffering. Although I might've argued with myself when life wasn't as easy, I know now that not looking as sick as you feel, and having some people not believe you, is *not* the hardest part of fibromyalgia. You are you and they are them. You must know what you know and understand that some people either don't want to or can't understand what you're going through.

Like any difficult situation, your attitude is the key. In this case, the glass can either be half empty or half full. Although some days I felt miserable and no one could tell, on a good day, I felt like a million bucks. And it was in this latter situation when not looking like the scourge of the Earth wasn't so bad.

So what about those who don't believe you? What about those who don't care enough to understand? Let's see, how do I put this? As my great grandfather used to say, in his thick Irish accent, "Ahhh meh-lad, meh-lad, dohn-cha werr-ee now. I would-na givem the steam ahf me pess."

Yes, my great grandfather was quite the philosopher. And not to be fooled with.

On the same general train of thought, recognize that no matter how well you engineer your daily life to cooperate with your body, you are going to have bad days. I feel great and I still have bad days. That's what fibromyalgia is. The trick is to have more good days than bad days, and if you are, you're already winning. Beyond that, there's not much more you can do. There is no cleansing process. You have fibromyalgia, and chances are you always will. But, take it from me, someone who was completely hopeless and cynical, that fibromyalgia is manageable.

Surround yourself with positive people and positive things. Nobody wants to hear how horrible it is to have fibromyalgia, and if you're anything like me, you don't want their pity anyway. Focus on positive things, find funny people and get each other laughing. No matter how bad you feel, I've always found you can still be the Moe to someone's Curly, the Costello to their Abbott, and the Daffy Duck to their Bugs Bunny. Strap on your Acme Rocket Skates, poke each other in the eyes ad nauseum, and enjoy the baseball game regardless of who's on first.

In conclusion, I *would* recommend getting closer to loving people who are funny and staying away from the nasty ones who are critical of everything you say and do.

CHAPTER 7

Endocrine Dysfunction Concurrent with Fibromyalgia

Sander J. Paul, MD

Could fibromyalgia be related to hypothyroidism and adrenal insufficiency? What about the speculation that fibromyalgia is unrecognized hypothyroidism or adrenal insufficiency? Is treatment with thyroid hormone or steroids recommended for fibromyalgia patients?

Let's look into these questions.

Thyroid Disease

The thyroid gland is a butterfly-shaped organ weighing slightly less than an ounce. It's in the lower neck below the Adam's apple and in front of the windpipe. The thyroid gland manufactures, stores, and releases two thyroid hormones, triiodothyronine (T3) and thyroxine

(T4). These hormones are made by combining iodine from the diet with the amino acid tyrosine. T3 has three iodine atoms per molecule, and T4 has four. All tissues in the body depend on thyroid hormone to regulate the cellular metabolism (chemical reactions) necessary for normal organ function.[1]

In the normal adult, the thyroid gland produces about 100 micrograms (mcg) of T4 daily. The daily production of T3 is about 30 mcg. About 20% (6 mcg) of T3 is secreted by the thyroid, and the rest is produced by the conversion of T4 to T3 in the peripheral tissues. Therefore, the thyroid gland secretes about 16 times as much T4 as T3.

T3 is the biologically active hormone with four times the potency of T4. T3 is rapidly and completely absorbed in the bloodstream, whereas T4 is slowly absorbed, and even then only about 80% of it is absorbed. Consequently, the blood level of T3 fluctuates, whereas the level of T4 remains fairly constant. The half-life of T4 in the bloodstream is one week (half-life is the time it takes for half the substance to be metabolized), whereas the half-life of T3 is one day.[1,2]

Two parts of the brain regulate the thyroid—the hypothalamus and the pituitary gland. These organs not only monitor the amount of T3 and T4 in the blood, but also the whole body's requirements for the hormones based on energy and metabolic needs. The hypothalamus secretes thyrotropin-releasing hormone (TRH), which stimulates the pituitary gland to secrete thyrotropin (thyroid stimulating hormone, or TSH). TSH signals the thyroid gland to manufacture, store, and release T3 and T4 into the bloodstream.[1] Refer to Figure 7.1.

Abnormal Thyroid Physiology

Hypothyroidism is a condition in which the thyroid gland produces too little thyroid hormone to maintain a healthy rate of metabolism. Hypothyroidism is not always a dysfunction of the gland itself; however, it is the problem 90–95% of the time. Hypothyroidism can also be caused when the hypothalamus or pituitary gland does not release enough TRH or TSH respectively. Hypothyroidism caused by a problem with the thyroid gland itself is called primary hypothyroidism; hypothyroidism caused by a problem with the brain's hypothalamus or pituitary gland is called central hypothyroidism.

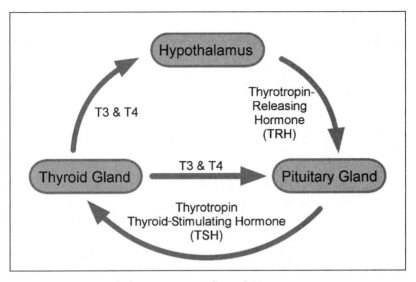

FIGURE 7.1   Hypothalamic-Pituitary-Thyroid Axis

Common causes of primary hypothyroidism include the following:

- Hashimoto's thyroiditis
- Radioactive iodine treatment for Graves' disease (hyperthyroidism)
- Thyroidectomy (removal of the thyroid gland, often for cancer)
- External radiation treatment to the neck for certain types of cancer
- Certain drugs such as lithium, amiodarone, and iodine

Causes of central hypothyroidism include pituitary tumors, head trauma, and head radiation for brain cancers.

Even rarer than primary and central hypothyroidism are thyroid-hormone resistance syndromes. Resistance to a hormone is defined as reduced or absent responsiveness to the hormone by the organs and tissues of the body. The tissues and organs don't respond to the hormone, and as a result, the hormone doesn't have the effect it should have. Resistance to thyroid hormone is caused by a mutation that affects the T3 receptor sites in cells' nuclei so that T3 cannot bind to cells' nuclei and cause its metabolic effects.[3,4,5]

Diagnosing Hypothyroidism

We base a diagnosis of hypothyroidism on a combination of things:

- A complete medical history
- A physical examination
- Laboratory tests

Important aspects of your medical history that increase the likelihood of hypothyroidism include:

- A family history of thyroid disease
- Previous neck surgery
- Previous treatment for hyperthyroidism with radioactive iodine therapy
- Treatment with drugs known to cause thyroid dysfunction

Suspicion of hypothyroidism is increased by hypothyroid symptoms (as discussed below) and the presence of other autoimmune diseases like adrenal insufficiency (Addison's disease), Type 1 diabetes mellitus, certain types of anemia, and vitiligo (loss of skin pigmentation). Important aspects of the physical examination include a slow pulse, an enlarged thyroid gland (goiter), and other signs as described below.[6]

Clinical manifestations of hypothyroidism are divided into two groups—those caused by slow metabolism and those caused by accumulation of abnormal cellular substances called matrix in the body's tissues. Symptoms caused by slow metabolism include fatigue, depression, memory loss, sleepiness, cold intolerance, weight gain, constipation, and a slow heart rate. Signs and symptoms caused by the accumulation of matrix in the tissues include hoarseness, dry and puffy skin, muscle weakness, joint aches, and fluid retention/weight gain.

This is by no means a complete listing of hypothyroidism's signs and symptoms. If you have fibromyalgia, you will recognize many of these symptoms as symptoms of fibromyalgia, too. Therefore, we must rule out hypothyroidism in fibromyalgia patients.[7,8]

Laboratory Diagnosis

Before we had reliable blood tests to measure thyroid hormones, we measured other things to infer thyroid hormone levels. For example, we measured serum cholesterol and CK muscle enzymes, which are higher in hypothyroidism. We measured oxygen consumption, which is lower in hypothyroidism. Basal body temperature is often used as a simple diagnostic tool, because it is low in hypothyroidism, but low body temperature doesn't necessarily mean you are hypothyroid. Similarly, the signs and symptoms noted above are often absent in patients with laboratory-proven hypothyroidism and are often present in patients without hypothyroidism.[6,9]

To confirm a diagnosis of hypothyroidism, we measure two things in laboratory blood tests: thyroid stimulating hormone (TSH) and free thyroxine (free T4).

The TSH test detects primary hypothyroidism. To understand the results, you need to understand how the pituitary and the thyroid work together. Let's take a moment to look at that.

Through TSH, the pituitary gland tells the thyroid gland when to speed up and when to slow down. How? The pituitary gland monitors the blood levels of T3 and T4. When these levels fall, it releases more TSH. The thyroid gland monitors the blood level of TSH. When it rises, the thyroid releases more T3 and T4. Of course, the opposite happens too: When the blood levels of T3 and T4 rise, the pituitary releases less TSH; when the blood level of TSH falls, the thyroid releases less T3 and T4.

Therefore, if something is wrong with the thyroid gland, the pituitary will keep trying to speed it up by releasing more and more TSH. Therefore, in patients with a sluggish thyroid gland, our blood tests show high TSH levels.

What's normal? I can give you numbers, but take them with a grain of salt, because test results depend on the test method used. But in many commercial assays, the normal range for TSH is 0.5–5.50 mU/L. Many people believe the target range for healthy individuals is 0.5–2.0 mU/L.[6,9,1]

When we test for how much thyroid hormone the thyroid gland is putting out, we test for free thyroxine. Free thyroxine is T4 not bound to blood proteins. Note that *free* thyroxine is but a small fraction of the total amount. Again, the normal range is laboratory-specific, but the usual range is 0.7–2.0 ng/dL. Typically, T4 levels begin to fall into the subnormal range after TSH has started to rise.

Other laboratory tests include total T3 and free T3 levels. These are not helpful in the diagnosis of hypothyroidism, because their levels often remain normal even after the free T4 begins to fall and long after TSH has begun to rise. The typical normal range for total T3 is 80–180 ng/dL. For free T3 it is 2.3–4.2 ng/ml.

We can also test for thyroid antibodies to detect evidence of autoimmune thyroid disease, such as Hashimoto's thyroiditis. In an autoimmune disease, the body produces antibodies that damage its own tissue cells. In this case, the damaging antibodies we find are antiperoxidase antibodies and antithyroglobulin antibodies, which attack normal thyroid cell components. The presence of one or both antibodies suggests either Hashimoto's thyroiditis or Graves' disease.[1,9]

Another laboratory test, which has historical importance, is the TRH test. As previously mentioned, the brain's hypothalamus releases TRH to tell the pituitary gland to release TSH. Therefore, a rise in TRH should be followed by a rise in TSH. The protocol for a TRH test:

1. Blood is drawn to measure a baseline TSH level.
2. The patient receives an intravenous injection of 250–500 mcg of TRH.
3. Fifteen-to-thirty minutes later, blood is drawn again to measure the effect of TRH on the TSH level.

In normal individuals, the TSH level rises from 2–20 mU/L above the baseline. An increase of more than 20 mU/L may represent early thyroid failure.

Some practitioners believe that the TRH test is the gold standard for diagnosing both primary and central hypothyroidism. But, because TSH testing is so accurate now, the TRH test has fallen out of favor and TRH is no longer available in the United States for diagnostic testing.[1]

Subclinical Hypothyroidism

Subclinical hypothyroidism is defined as a normal free T4 level and a mildly elevated TSH level (5–15 mU/L). Patients with subclinical hypothyroidism cannot be identified by signs or symptoms.

The causes of subclinical hypothyroidism are the same as the causes of primary hypothyroidism. Subclinical hypothyroidism occurs in about 15% of women over the age of 65, in 8% of men over age 65, and in 2% of pregnant women. A significant percentage of people with subclinical hypothyroidism will eventually develop symptomatic (overt) hypothyroidism, at a rate of 4–8% per year. Those with the highest baseline TSH levels and those with thyroid antibodies progress the most rapidly to overt hypothyroidism.

If the TSH level is greater than 10 mU/L, the current recommendation for treatment is thyroid hormone replacement. For subclinical hypothyroid patients with a TSH between 5 and 10 mU/L, the benefit of this treatment is less certain, and whether to treat should be discussed with the patient. Note, however, that all pregnant patients with a TSH greater than 5 mU/L should be treated with thyroid hormone.[10] See Figure 7.2.

Treating Hypothyroidism

The goal of treatment is to restore the tissue levels of thyroid hormone to normal and thus resolve the signs and symptoms of hypothyroidism. We usually achieve this goal by administering thyroxine pills in a dose high enough to do two things:

- Restore the TSH level to within the normal range
- Restore the free T4 level to within the normal range

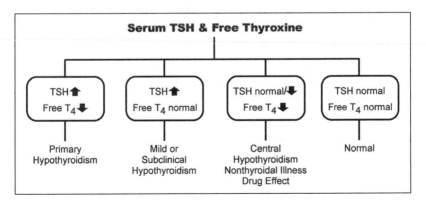

FIGURE 7.2   Diagnosis of thyroid disorders based on: serum TSH & free thyroxine

Of course, in patients with central hypothyroidism (in which TSH secretion is abnormal), the TSH levels are an invalid indicator, so we must rely solely on the free T4 levels to monitor treatment.[2,11]

Dosing

We base your initial dose of thyroxine (T4) on your age, your general health, and the severity of your hypothyroidism. In healthy adults, a full replacement dose is approximately 1.6 micrograms per kilogram of body weight per day. The usual replacement dose is between 75 and 150 mcg daily. In older individuals with heart disease, we start lower and go slower in increasing doses, to reduce the risk of angina (cardiac chest pain).

Ideally, you take T4 upon arising, with water only, and you wait an hour before eating, drinking, or taking other prescription medications. Normally the body absorbs 80% of the T4 in the pill you take, but over-the-counter medications (especially calcium, iron, and multivitamins) may reduce absorption to less than 50% so avoid taking these with your T4.[2,11]

Synthetic T4, or levothyroxine, is manufactured in both branded and generic tablets. In 2004, the Food and Drug Administration (FDA) approved generic substitutions for branded levothyroxine products. The thyroid-specialty physician associations opposed this decision, and I also recommend that patients remain on the branded (Synthroid, Levothroid, Levoxyl, and Unithroid) products. If you change brands or switch to generics, your TSH level should be assessed 6 to 8 weeks later. The concern with generics is that pharmacies may frequently change their generic levothyroxine manufacturer without notifying the patient, potentially affecting their thyroid hormone balance.

Monitoring Therapy

After therapy begins, it takes weeks for the body to adjust and establish a new, steady TSH level. Therefore, in 6 to 8 weeks (no earlier), your TSH and free T4 levels should be checked and your prescription dosage adjusted accordingly. Increases (or decreases) in dosage should be limited to 25 mcg/day. The target range for TSH is 0.5–2.0 mU/L in healthy individuals successfully treated with levothyroxine.

The appropriate levothyroxine dosage should normalize levels of TSH and free T4, as well as resolve the signs and symptoms of hypothyroidism. Because tissue levels take longer to return to normal than blood levels, these signs and symptoms may persist until 3 months after TSH normalizes. At that point we know the optimum dose for you.

Nonetheless, your TSH level should be reassessed every 6 to 12 months—more frequently if there is a significant change in your clinical status due to such things as pregnancy, marked weight change, or surgery.[2,11]

Treating Hypothyroidism in Fibromyalgia Patients

There is a significant controversy in the fibromyalgia literature as to whether fibromyalgia is caused by unrecognized hypothyroidism. The fibromyalgia consensus committees[12] suggest that fibromyalgia and hypothyroidism are concurrent conditions with different causes. Since fibromyalgia and hypothyroidism occur in young females, and because the symptoms overlap considerably, it is important to screen all fibromyalgia patients for hypothyroidism.

For example, if a 30-year-old woman with fibromyalgia complains of diffuse muscle pains, fatigue, depression, and poor memory, I would thoroughly evaluate her for hypothyroidism by history, physical exam, and laboratory studies. If this young woman had a family history of thyroid disease, a goiter, thyroid antibodies, and a TSH of 4.0 mU/L, I would treat her with levothyroxine, even though her TSH falls within the "normal" range. If her previous TSH levels are available, they might show a previous TSH in the 1.0–2.0 mU/L range, suggesting that she has early Hashimoto's thyroiditis and impending thyroid failure. My hope would be that early treatment with levothyroxine significantly improves her symptoms of fibromyalgia/hypothyroidism.

On the other hand, the same 30-year-old woman with no family history, no goiter, no thyroid antibodies, and a TSH of 2.0 mU/L isn't hypothyroid. Yet some fibromyalgia researchers feel that she has "euthyroid" fibromyalgia—fibromyalgia with hypothyroid symptoms but normal blood levels of TSH. They believe such patients have a form of thyroid hormone resistance and should be treated with large doses of triiodothyronine (T3), ranging from 94 to 225 mcg. Of course, the pituitary will react by reducing output of TSH to low levels, so low as to be undetectable in blood tests.[13] I'll discuss T3 therapy and TSH suppression later.

To treat a fibromyalgia patient with hypothyroidism, I prescribe a branded, synthetic T4 and adjust the dosage to attain a TSH level of 0.5–2.0 mU/L. My experience with patients who have both fibromyalgia and hypothyroidism is that attaining this goal often fails to produce a normal sense of well-being. This may be due to the overlap of symptoms between the two diseases or to unrealistic expectations of the treatment's benefits.

T3 Therapy

If the patient with both hypothyroidism and fibromyalgia continues to complain of symptoms that are possibly due to hypothyroidism despite a levothyroxine (T4) dose that normalizes TSH, then I consider T3 replacement therapy.

Available Products

Many products on the market contain T4 and T3. Natural thyroid products are those extracted from the thyroid glands of pigs. They contain both T4 and T3. Brand names include Armour thyroid, Naturethroid, and Westhroid. Natural thyroid has a T4 to T3 ratio of 3:1. Recall that the normal human thyroid secretes a 16:1 ratio of T4 to T3. Therefore, natural thyroid has too much T3 to serve as a good replacement. Liotrex (brand name Thyrolar) is another T3/T4 product. It's a synthetic combination of T4 and T3 in a ratio of 4:1. It also has too much T3. A synthetic T3 (triiodothyronine) compound (brand name Cytomel) is also available in strengths of 5 mcg, 25 mcg, and 50 mcg.[2]

Controversies

The use of T3 in combination with T4 to treat hypothyroidism is controversial. There are drawbacks to T3 therapy: Its short half-life and its rapid, complete absorption result in unstable T3 blood levels, with much of the day spent at above normal T3 blood levels. The patient may feel palpitations because of these high T3 levels.

To date, there have been eight randomized trials using combinations of T3 and T4. Only the initial study showed improvement in mood and neuropsychologic function when 12.5 mcg of T3 was substituted for 50 mcg of T4 (i.e., a patient on 125 mcg of T4 would be converted to 12.5 mcg of T3 and 75 mcg of T4).[14] Seven subsequent studies with varying substitution protocols failed to show a significant improvement in cognitive function, mood, well-being, and quality of life.[11,15]

My Approach

Despite the conflicting data on T3 and T4 combination replacement therapies, I offer the patient with hypothyroidism and fibromyalgia a trial of combined therapy, if they remain symptomatic on thyroxine alone with a goal TSH level. I try to mimic the normal thyroid gland production ratio of 100 mcg per day of T4 and 6 mcg per day of T3 (a 16:1 ratio).

For patients on a T4 dose between 50 and 125 mcg, I say to continue the same T4 dose, but to skip one day a week and to add 5 mcg of Cytomel daily. For example, if a patient is taking 100 mcg of T4 daily, I reduce the dose to 100 mcg six days a week and add Cytomel 5 mcg daily.

For patients on a T4 dose at 150 mcg or more, I say to continue the same T4 dose but only six days a week and to add Cytomel at a dose of 5% of their starting T4 dose. For example, if a patient is taking 200 mcg of T4 daily, reduce the dose to 200 mcg six days a week and add 10 mcg (200 mcg × 0.05) of Cytomel daily.

These regimens are designed to maintain the normal thyroid T4 to T3 ratio of 16:1 and the fourfold increased potency of T3 over T4.

I recheck TSH, free T4 and free T3 levels 6 to 8 weeks after conversion to assess the adequacy of the dosages, and adjust as necessary. I generally wait 3 to 4 months after confirmed normal thyroid levels to decide if continuing the T3/T4 combination has truly improved symptoms. In my experience with this regimen, about three out of four patients with both hypothyroidism and fibromyalgia demonstrate significant improvement in symptoms and an increased feeling of well-being.

Subclinical Hyperthyroidism

Finally, I want to address the concern that endocrinologists have about the risk of excessive thyroid hormone consumption—that is, *hyperthyroidism* caused by excessive T3 and/or T4 intake.

If excessive T3 and/or T4 is taken regularly, TSH levels fall, often to an undetectable level, and serum T3 and T4 levels may rise above their normal ranges. Commonly, I see patients with TSH levels in the 0.05 to 0.5 mU/L range, who have normal T3 and T4 levels and no symptoms of hyperthyroidism (subclinical hyperthyroidism). Some practitioners believe that every fibromyalgia patient has unrecognized hypothyroidism, even those with clearly normal TSH and T4 levels. Such patients are often treated with large doses of T3 (as discussed earlier), suppressing TSH to an undetectable level, and often raising T3 levels to two to four times the upper limit of the normal range.[13]

Whereas it is clear that *overt* hyperthyroidism (elevated T3 and/or T4 levels with undetectable TSH levels) can cause osteoporosis and increase the risk of hip and vertebral fractures, the skeletal effects of *subclinical* hyperthyroidism are less clear. There have been studies in which bone mineral density was measured in the hip and spine in T4 treated patients with suppressed TSH levels. From these studies, it appears that postmenopausal women are at risk for decreased bone density and perhaps increased fracture risk. But little decrease in bone density is seen in premenopausal women. The other major concern in patients with subclinical hyperthyroidism is atrial fibrillation, especially in older individuals, which can lead to strokes. It is important to discuss the risks associated with subclinical hyperthyroidism and to adjust the thyroid hormone dose to return the TSH to a more normal range.[10(pp1079–1085),16,17,18]

Adrenal Disease

The adrenal glands are pyramid-shaped structures draping above the upper pole of each kidney, each weighing about one fifth of an ounce. The adrenal gland is composed of an outer layer of tissue called the adrenal cortex (90% of the adrenal gland's weight) and an inner layer called the adrenal medulla. The cortex produces the hormones cortisol and aldosterone, as well as sex hormones; the medulla produces adrenaline (epinephrine).

Cortisol's most important role is to help the body respond to stress. In addition to its many other roles, it helps maintain blood pressure and heart function, it slows the immune system's inflammatory activity, and it helps metabolize nutrients. Aldosterone helps maintain blood pressure and the body's water-and-salt balance.

Like the thyroid gland, the adrenal cortex is regulated by the hypothalamus and the pituitary gland. These organs monitor the blood levels of cortisol and aldosterone, as well as the body's requirement for these hormones based on your salt-and-water balance, blood pressure, physical stress, and emotional stress. The hypothalamus secretes corticotropin-releasing hormone (CRH) which stimulates the pituitary gland to secrete corticotropin (adrenocorticotropin hormone, or ACTH). ACTH stimulates the adrenal cortex to manufacture, store, and release cortisol and aldosterone.[19,20]

Abnormal Adrenal Physiology

Hypoadrenalism or adrenal ("adrenocortical") insufficiency (AI) is a condition in which the body produces too little cortisol and/or aldosterone. Primary AI (due to damaged adrenal glands) is rare, whereas secondary AI (due to a problem with the hypothalamus or pituitary) is common.

Common causes of primary adrenal insufficiency include autoimmune adrenalitis (Addison's disease, which accounts for 70–80% of all cases of primary AI), infections (e.g., tuberculosis, fungi, HIV), adrenal hemorrhage (from blood thinners or bacterial toxins), bilateral adrenalectomy (removal of both adrenal glands, usually for cancer), and certain drugs. The most common cause of secondary adrenal insufficiency is tapering off a steroid drug too quickly or premature cessation of steroids given for other medical problems such as asthma or rheumatism. Less common causes of secondary AI include pituitary tumors, head trauma, and radiation treatment of the head for brain cancer.[19,20]

Diagnosing Adrenal Insufficiency

We base a diagnosis of adrenal insufficiency on a combination of things:

- A complete medical history
- A physical exam
- Laboratory testing

Important aspects of your medical history that increase the likelihood of AI include the use of oral, topical, rectal, or inhaled steroids in the previous six months. Suspicion of AI is increased by hypoadrenal symptoms (as discussed below) and the presence of autoimmune disease (Hashimoto's thyroiditis, Graves' disease, Type 1 diabetes mellitus, hypoparathyroidism, anemia, and vitiligo). Important aspects of the physical exam include weight loss, low blood pressure, hyperpigmentation (darkening of the skin), and vitiligo.[19,20]

Clinical manifestations of adrenal insufficiency differ in primary and secondary AI. Patients with primary AI have (1) low cortisol and aldosterone levels and (2) a high ACTH level, which causes hyperpigmentation of skin in areas exposed to the sun. Patients with secondary AI have a low cortisol level, a normal aldosterone level, and a low ACTH level. So, they have no hyperpigmentation, and their electrolyte disorders (water-and-salt imbalances) are less severe. Symptoms common to both primary and secondary AI include weakness, fatigue, anorexia, weight loss, low blood pressure, muscle and joint pain, and gastrointestinal complaints like nausea and vomiting. Vitiligo and salt craving are seen only in primary AI.

This is by no means a complete listing of adrenal insufficiency's signs and symptoms. If you have fibromyalgia, you recognize many of these signs and symptoms as signs and symptoms of fibromyalgia, too. Therefore, we must rule out adrenal insufficiency in fibromyalgia patients.[19,20]

Laboratory Diagnosis

Common blood abnormalities include low sodium, high potassium (in primary AI), high calcium, and low glucose. Unfortunately, a single measurement of cortisol and ACTH isn't sensitive enough to be diagnostic. So, patients should undergo an ACTH stimulation test. Normal morning levels of ACTH and cortisol are laboratory specific, because they depend on the method and equipment used. But, as a rule, early morning ACTH levels are 5–45 pg/ml and cortisol levels are 5–25 mcg/dl.[19,20]

The ACTH stimulation test (also called Cortrosyn or Cosyntropin stimulation test) follows this procedure:

1. Blood is drawn to measure its baseline serum ACTH and cortisol levels.
2. The patient receives an intravenous or intramuscular injection of 250 mcg of synthetic ACTH (Cortrosyn).
3. Thirty minutes after injection, blood is drawn again to measure the effect of ACTH on the cortisol level.
4. Sixty minutes after injection, blood is drawn yet again to measure the cortisol level.

A normal response to the injection of ACTH is defined as a peak level of cortisol greater than 20 mcg/dl. Because there are limitations to this test, other more complex diagnostic tests for AI are available, but they are beyond the scope of this chapter.[19,20] Yet, the ACTH stimulation test is excellent for screening people with chronic symptoms. (By "chronic" symptoms, I mean symptoms persisting longer than 2 months.)

For example, a 40-year-old woman with fibromyalgia fatigue, weight loss, and muscle aches, who looked like she has a summer tan in February, has the following results:

- *Baseline ACTH level:* 350 pg/ml (normal is 5–45 pg/ml)
- *Baseline cortisol level:* 4 mcg/dl
- *Thirty-minute cortisol level:* 7 mcg/dl
- *Sixty-minute cortisol level:* 6 mcg/dl

These results would suggest this woman has primary AI concurrent with fibromyalgia.

Treating Adrenal Insufficiency

The goal of treatment is to restore the tissue levels of cortisol and aldosterone to normal and thus resolve the signs and symptoms of AI. We usually achieve this goal by administering hydrocortisone pills in a dosage of 20–30 mg/day split into two or three doses (breakfast and dinner, or breakfast, lunch, and dinner). For aldosterone replacement in primary AI, you need Florinef (9 alpha fludrocortisone) in a dose of 0.05–0.2 mg/day daily at breakfast.

We base decisions about dosages on the clinical signs and symptoms, a return to normal weight and blood pressure, less fatigue, less anorexia, and less joint and muscle pain.

Unfortunately, there is no reliable blood or urine test to confirm the perfect dose. Because of concerns about osteoporosis from hydrocortisone and fluid retention from fludrocortisone, patients should take the lowest effective dose of both steroids, and they should be taught how to increase their hydrocortisone dose when under physical stress. They should also wear a medical alert bracelet or necklace for adrenal insufficiency.[19,20]

Treating Adrenal Insufficiency in Fibromyalgia Patients

There is significant controversy in the fibromyalgia literature as to whether fibromyalgia is caused by unrecognized adrenal insufficiency. One hypothesis is that fibromyalgia patients have altered brain function that alters pain processing by the hypothalamic-pituitary-adrenal axis and the autonomic nervous system. The fatigue, sleep disturbances, myalgias, gastrointestinal complaints, and impaired cognitive function may be due to misalignment of the internal biological clock with abnormal sleep–wake cycles.

But clinical studies of fibromyalgia patients show normal circadian rhythms and normal diurnal cortisol and melatonin levels during the day and night. In addition, the hypothalamic-pituitary-adrenal axis of fibromyalgia patients has been tested by inducing hypoglycemia through insulin injection. Hypoglycemia creates severe physiological stress, which activates the axis. Fibromyalgia patients respond with slightly lower ACTH levels than others do, but their cortisol response to stress is normal.

Nonetheless, the slightly lower levels of ACTH that fibromyalgia patients respond with is intriguing and may represent reduced signaling from the hypothalamus to the pituitary.[21,22]

Hydrocortisone Therapy

Numerous studies have sought to learn whether steroid therapy is helpful to patients with fibromyalgia and chronic fatigue syndrome. A

2-week study of prednisone at 15 mg/day showed no improvement in symptoms. Hydrocortisone at 25–35 mg/day for 3 months showed some improvement in well-being but no improvement in fatigue, and patients experienced side effects including weight gain and adrenal suppression. About a third of people treated with low-dose cortisol at 5–10 mg/day for one month reported a decrease in fatigue.

Given the general lack of improvement and the side effects (including weight gain, bone loss, sleep disturbances, and adrenal gland suppression), steroid therapy isn't recommended for fibromyalgia patients with normal Cortrosyn stimulation test results.[21]

My Approach

In the rare patient with both adrenal insufficiency and fibromyalgia, I try to establish whether the AI is primary or secondary. I treat with hydrocortisone and fludrocortisone as discussed earlier. I have patients who I think were inappropriately given steroids for fibromyalgia symptoms and who now have steroid-induced secondary AI. It is very difficult to wean these patients from steroids, because the symptoms of steroid withdrawal overlap with the symptoms of fibromyalgia, making it tough for fibromyalgia patients to taper off steroids. In my experience, it's imperative to taper off slowly and steadily, running ACTH stimulation tests to assess recovery of the pituitary-adrenal axis.

Conclusions

- Patients with fibromyalgia have clinical signs and symptoms that overlap with both hypothyroidism and adrenal insufficiency. It is therefore imperative to rule out these two endocrine disorders.
- I don't believe that all patients with fibromyalgia suffer from unrecognized hypothyroidism or unrecognized adrenal insufficiency that cannot be diagnosed with routine endocrine testing.
- In fibromyalgia patients with documented hypothyroidism or adrenal insufficiency, the goals of therapy are to restore tissue hormone levels to normal and relieve the signs and symptoms of the disorder.

- In patients with both hypothyroidism and fibromyalgia, I often use combinations of thyroxine and triiodothyronine to try to restore the balance of T3 and T4 normally produced in the thyroid gland.
- In patients with both adrenal insufficiency and fibromyalgia, I use combinations of hydrocortisone and fludrocortisone to try to restore the balance of cortisol and aldosterone normally produced by the adrenal glands.

References

1. Utiger RD. The thyroid: physiology, thyrotoxicosis, hypothyroidism and the painful thyroid. In: Felig P, Frohman L, eds. *Endocrinology and Metabolism.* 4th ed. New York, NY: McGraw-Hill; 2001:261-347.
2. Woeber KA. Treatment of hypothyroidism. In: Braverman L, Utiger L, eds. *Werner & Ingbar's The Thyroid: A Fundamental and Clinical Text.* 9th ed. Philadelphia, PA: Lippincott Williams & Wilkins; 2005: 864-869.
3. Braverman LE, Utiger RD. Introduction to hypothyroidism. In: Braverman L, Utiger R, eds. *Werner & Ingbar's The Thyroid: A Fundamental and Clinical Text.* 9th ed. Philadelphia, PA: Lippincott Williams & Wilkins; 2005:697-699.
4. Ross DS. Disorders that cause hypothyroidism. UpToDate online version 13.1. Available at: http://www.uptodate.com. Accessed October 30, 2006.
5. Ross DS. Resistance to thyroid hormone, thyrotropin, and thyrotropin-releasing hormone. UpToDate online version 13.1. Available at: http://www.uptodate.com. Accessed October 30, 2006.
6. Ladenson PW. Managment of hypothyroidism. In: Braverman L, Utiger L, eds. *Werner & Ingbar's The Thyroid: A Fundamental and Clinical Text.* 9th ed. Philadelphia, PA: Lippincott Williams & Wilkins; 2005:857-863.
7. Braverman LE, Utiger RD. Introduction to hypothyroidism. In: Braverman L, Utiger R, eds. *Werner & Ingbar's The Thyroid: A Fundamental and Clinical Text.* 9th ed. Philadelphia, PA: Lippincott Williams & Wilkins; 2005:697-699.
8. Ross DS. Diagnosis of and screening for hypothyroidism. UpToDate online version 13.1. Available at: http://www.uptodate.com. Accessed October 30, 2006.

9. Ross DS. Laboratory assessment of thyroid function. UpToDate online version 13.1. Available at: http://www.uptodate.com. Accessed October 30, 2006.

10. Ross DS. Subclinical hypothyroidism. In: Braverman L, Utiger R, eds. *Werner & Ingbar's The Thyroid: A Fundamental and Clinical Text.* 9th ed. Philadelphia, PA: Lippincott Williams & Wilkins; 2005:1070-1078.

11. Ross DS. Treatment of hypothyroidism. UpToDate online version 13.1. Available at: http://www.uptodate.com. Accessed October 30, 2006.

12. Wolfe F, Smythe HA, Yunus MB, et al. The American college of rehumatology 1990 criteria for the classification of fibromyalgia: report of the multicenter criteria committee. *Arthritis Rheum.* 1990;33:160-172.

13. Garrison RL, Breeding PC. A metabolic basis for fibromyalgia and its related disorders: the possible role of resistance to thyroid hormone. *Med Hypotheses.* 2003;61(2):182-189.

14. Bunnevicius R, Kazanavicus G, Zalinkevicius R, et al. Effects of thyroxine as compared with thyroxine plus triiodothyronine in patients with hypothyroidism. *N Engl J Med.* 1999:424-429.

15. Utiger RD, ed. *Clinical Thyroidology.* 2005;17(2):29-31.

16. Franklyn JA, Gammage MD. Morbidity and mortality in thyroid dysfunction and its treatment. In: Braverman L, Utiger R, eds. *Werner & Ingbar's The Thyroid: A Fundamental and Clinical Text.* 9th ed. Philadelphia, PA: Lippincott Williams & Wilkins; 2005:1063-1078.

17. Ross DS. Bone disease with hyperthyroidism and thyroid hormone therapy. UpToDate online version 13.1. Available at: http://www. uptodate.com. Accessed October 30, 2006.

18. Shepard MC, Gittoes, NJL. The skeletal system in thyrotoxicosis. In: Braverman L, Utiger R, eds. *Werner & Ingbar's The Thyroid: A Fundamental and Clinical Text.* 9th ed. Philadelphia, PA: Lippincott Williams & Wilkins; 2005:629-636.

19. Miller WL, Chrousos GP. The adrenal cortex. In: Felig P, Frohman L, eds. *Endocrinology and Metabolism.* 4th ed. New York, NY: McGraw-Hill; 2001:387-524.

20. Stewart PM. The adrenal cortex. In: Larson PR, Kronenberg H, Melmed S, eds. *Williams Textbook of Endocrinology.* 10th ed. Philadelphia, PA: Saunders; 2003:491-551.

21. Adler GK. HPA Axis and Fatigue. Presented at the 2005 Endocrine Society Meeting; June, 2005; San Diego, CA.

22. Adler GK, Kinsley B, Hurwitz S, et al. Reduced hypothalamic-pituitary and sypathoadrenal responses to hypoglycemia in women with fibromyalgia syndrome. *Am J Med.* 1999;106:534-543.

CHAPTER 8

Temporomandibular Disorders (TMD) and Facial Pain

Ghabi Kaspo, D.D.S.

The symptoms of temporomandibular dysfunction (TMD) include pain and dysfunction in the head, neck, face, and jaw. These symptoms are often multiple and varied.

If you think you may be suffering from TMD, here are a few questions you can ask yourself. However, keep in mind that a reliable diagnosis can't be based solely on your answers to these questions. "Yes" answers just let you know that you or someone you know should seek professional advice.

- Do you hear popping, clicking, or cracking sounds when you chew?
- Do your jaws feel like they "catch"?

- Do your ears hurt?
- Do your jaws ache after eating?
- Does it seem like you cannot open your mouth as wide as you used to?
- Do you hear a grating sound (like crumpling newspaper) when you chew?
- Does it hurt to move your jaw open and sideways?
- Do you have stuffiness, pressure, or blockage in your ears?
- Do you hear a ringing or buzzing in either or both of your ears?
- Do you wake with sore facial muscles?
- Do you have frequent headaches?
- Do you experience dizziness frequently?
- Do your jaws feel tight and hard to open?
- Does your tongue go between your teeth, or do you bite on your tongue to separate your teeth?
- Do your teeth ache, and are they sensitive to cold?
- Do you clench or grind your teeth when frustrated or concentrating?
- Do you grind your teeth at night?
- Does your neck, the back of your head, or your shoulder hurt?
- Have you been hit in the jaw?
- Have you been put to sleep for surgery?
- Have you had a whiplash injury?
- Have you seen a neurologist, chiropractor, psychologist, or psychiatrist for unexplained head or neck pain?
- Are you under a lot of stress?

If you answered "Yes" to any of the questions on the list, you might be suffering with some form of TMD. The more "Yes" answers, the greater the odds of it.

The rest of this chapter will tell you about TMD, giving you background information and discussing both the diagnosis and management options for TMD.

Musculoskeletal Disorders

TMD is a musculoskeletal disorder, which means that it affects muscles and bones. Sometimes people refer to TMD as TMJ, the correct term, as recommended by the American Dental Association, is TMD, or temporomandibular disorders.

Musculoskeletal disorders are the most prevalent cause of chronic health problems, disabilities, and health care utilization. They are the second most common reason for restricting activity and consuming medication.[1]

Temporomandibular disorders are *not* adequately recognized by the medical community and *are* reported by a large proportion of fibromyalgia patients. Both TMD and fibromyalgia affect the muscles of the face, head, neck, shoulders, and back. Unfortunately, both TMD and fibromyalgia often go undiagnosed.

Eighty-five percent of people who suffer from fibromyalgia also suffer from TMD. We see the disorder most frequently in women between the ages of 20 and 50. In 1993 I studied 400 TMD patients and found that 5–6% of them had symptoms similar to fibromyalgia symptoms.[2,3]

TMJ Anatomy

TMJ is an abbreviation for the *temporomandibular joint*, which is the jaw joint. The temporomandibular joint connects the lower jaw, called the mandible (6), to the temporal bone (5) on the side of the head. If you place your fingers just in front of your ears and open your mouth, you can feel this joint on each side of your head. Because these joints are flexible, the jaw can move smoothly up and down and side to side, enabling us to talk, chew, and yawn. Muscles attached to, and surrounding, the jaw joint control its position and movement. Refer to Figure 8.1 for a side view of the Temporomandibular Joint.

When we open our mouths, the rounded ends of the lower jaw, called condyles (1), glide along the joint socket of the temporal bone. The condyles slide back to their original position when we close our mouths. To keep this motion smooth, a soft disc (3) lies between the condyle and the temporal bone. This disc absorbs shocks to the TMJ from chewing and other movements.

The two bones of the TMJ are held together by a series of ligaments, any of which can be damaged, just like the ligaments of any other joint. A damaged TMJ ligament usually results in dislocation of the disc, looseness of the mandible (lower jaw), or both.

Also, two main muscles connect the mandible and the temporal bone: the temporalis and the masseter. Either muscle may be painful, and either may produce pain in the TMJ or abnormal movement of the lower jaw.

The nerve to the TMJ is a branch of the trigeminal nerve. One TMJ can't function without affecting the other one, so if one TMJ is injured, the other joint will usually be affected some time in the future. This is true for knees and ankles as well.

Injured ligaments rarely completely heal, and this is especially true of TMJ ligaments. Some are extremely small. The powerful forces exerted on them by frequent chewing make proper healing nearly impossible.

To accommodate such frequent use and to help us open our mouths wide, the TMJ has two motions. The first movement is the hinging movement; the second movement is the sliding, or translation, movement within the socket of the temporal bone.[4]

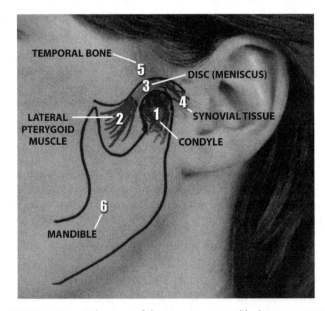

FIGURE 8.1   Side view of the Temporomandibular Joint (TMJ)

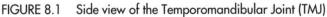

Muscles Associated with the TMJs

There are many muscles in the head, neck, and face associated with the TMJs. In fact, virtually all muscles of the neck, back, throat, and face directly or indirectly affect the TMJs.

Chewing Muscles Associated with TMD

Both the temporalis (1) and masseter (2) are powerful muscles, capable together of applying as much as 750–1,000 pounds of pressure on the teeth! All these chewing muscles are paired: there is one on the right side and one on the left. Refer to Figure 8.2.

Lightly press your fingers against the sides of your face, just below the cheeks, and clench your teeth. Do you feel the masseter muscles (2) bulging? Often, these muscles become sore after clenching, grinding, or an injury to the TMJ. The masseter muscles can become enlarged when they are overused over a long period of time. The masseter muscles close the lower jaw and aid in chewing.

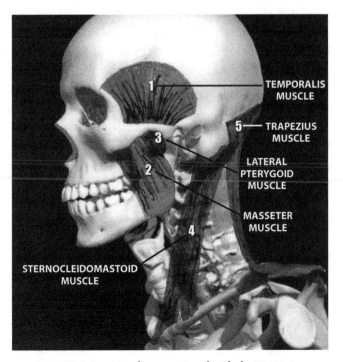

FIGURE 8.2   Muscles associated with the TMJ joint

Locate the temporalis (1) muscle by pushing against your temples and then clench your teeth. Feel the temporalis muscles bulging? That is the anterior belly of the temporalis muscles. The temporalis muscles close the mouth and draw the jaw backwards, helping us chew efficiently.

Neck Muscles Associated with TMD

We often see patients with their head thrust forward and their chin tilted up. This usually occurs in those who have a small lower jaw or who have had a neck injury. This posture also happens in those who sit for hours at a computer or typewriter.

Forward head posture causes the mandible to close differently than it should, thus causing malocclusion (bad bite). This in turn may make people grind or clench their teeth. This forward head posture also causes tension in the muscles of the neck and back, producing head, neck, and back pain. Frequently, these painful muscles refer pain into the head, face, and TMJs, causing both patient and doctor to think that the pain is coming from the TMJs. Can you see how confusing the process of diagnosing pain can be?

The names of the neck and back muscles are unimportant. However, the effect from increased tension in these muscles is important. Muscles work against each other in opposing pairs, so tension in some disturbs the dynamic balance of the whole system. If this imbalance continues for any length of time, we can experience head, facial, and TMJ pain without these structures really being physically injured.

Symptoms of TMD

Today, clinicians agree that temporomandibular disorders fall into three main categories:

- Muscle pain
- Internal derangement of the joint
- Degenerative joint disease

Let's look at each.

Muscle Pain

Probably the primary source of pain in TMD is muscle pain. Muscle pain arises from the muscles and the fascia, which are sheaths that surround the muscles. There are several different hypotheses about the exact mechanisms for how muscles become painful; however, most investigators agree that muscles can become inflamed, which causes increased temperature over the entire muscle. In addition the muscles can become swollen following severe sustained muscle contraction.

Internal Derangement of the TMJ

Internal derangements of the TMJ are disturbances in the arrangement of the components within the joint itself, primarily the disc. Internal derangement is the most common disorder of the TMJ.

There are many types of internal derangements of the TMJ. The most common is a clicking joint. Another is a locking joint, which could intermittently lock or permanently lock.

Derangements occur in all joints. The difference with the TMJ is that the joint's disc actually moves with normal jaw movement, acting like a third bone.

In the clicking joint (an anterior dislocation of the disc), the disc slips forward with a subsequent posterior displacement of the condyle. So, as the mouth opens, a "click" occurs when the disc gets caught between the bones. This catching of the disc between the bones isn't always heard, but it can be felt.

During intermittent locking the patient feels the jaw catch for a few seconds or minutes, but he or she can manipulate the jaw and open wider after a click.

In permanent locking, it may feel like the lower jaw is locked shut, and the patient cannot open it beyond a certain point. Sometimes a person with a locked jaw must move it to one side or the other to open wide, at which point the jaw mercifully unlocks. In most instances, the locking is painful.

The TMJ may lock open, as well. When that happens, the jaw is dislocated out of the socket. This is a terrifying experience. It usually occurs after a wide opening movement such as a yawn. However, an open lock can also occur after a long dental appointment in which the mouth is opened wide without using a bite block, or after being put to sleep for any type of surgery, or even after opening wide to eat an apple or large sandwich. Open locking that occurs repeatedly is a sign of weak or loose TMJ ligaments. We often see this in teenage girls limber enough to perform as cheerleaders or gymnasts.[5]

Degenerative Joint Disease

Examples of degenerative joint disease associated with TMD are osteoarthritis or rheumatoid arthritis in the jaw joint. A person may have one or more of these conditions at the same time. In addition, the bones can become thin and brittle, as in the case of osteoporosis. The bone thinning can lead to premature tooth loss when it occurs in the context of TMD.

Additional Symptoms Associated with TMD

Because TMD has so many symptoms, making a proper diagnosis is difficult. However, there are a few classic symptoms that involve the TM joints, ears, head, face, and teeth.

Ear Discomfort

Due to the close relationship of the TMJs and ears, an injury to the TMJ often causes ear symptoms. That is why many TMD sufferers first go to their family doctor and then to an ear doctor for help. Some of the symptoms are pain, fullness or stuffiness, and even a loss of hearing. Usually, an examination of the ear is normal, even if there appears to be a loss of hearing. Often the primary care physician puts the patient on antibiotic medication for a while, especially if the symptoms occur in the winter, even in the absence of other symptoms that usually signal an infection (fever, redness, heat, discharge).

Headache

Headache is one of the most common symptoms of a TMJ problem. Usually, the TMJ headache is in the temples, the back of the head, and even the shoulders. Clenching and grinding the teeth, both of which themselves may be TMD symptoms, produce muscle pain, which can cause headache pain. Also, a displaced disc in the TMJ may cause pain in the joint that is often referred into the temples, forehead, or neck. These headaches are frequently so severe that they are confused and treated as migraine headaches or abnormalities in the brain.

If a patient has seen many doctors and therapists, has taken all types of medication, has tried all sorts of exercises, and still has headache pain, then a TMD problem should be highly suspected. These unfortunate patients have often had many X-rays, CAT scans, and MRIs, yet no diagnosis. And worse, they continue to suffer.

Facial Pain

When we hurt, our faces show pain, although TMD may be referred to the face even though the TMJ itself does not really hurt. Facial pain may be deep in the face or on the surface. The skin might even become sensitive to the touch or air blowing over it.

TMD patients may experience pain in and behind the eye, which can cause sensitivity to light. Blurred vision and eye muscle twitching are also common in TMD patients.

Teeth Clenching

Severe teeth clenching may cause tooth pain and sensitivity. The teeth may become sensitive to temperature, especially cold. Patients may see their dentist for pain in the teeth, but the dentist can find no cause. Frequently (and unfortunately), unnecessary root canals and even tooth extractions are performed in an attempt to help a suffering person. What's worse, after these invasive and nonreversible procedures, patients still have their pain, only now it has increased!

Depression

Depression is common with TMD, as it is with all severe chronic pain conditions. Along with depression comes an inability to get a good night's sleep. Sufferers often awake feeling as though they never slept. This lack of sleep not only makes their pain worse, but also adds fuel to the fire of depression.

Referred Sensory Phenomena

Referred sensory phenomena (RSP) include sensory phenomena and autonomic phenomena. RSP involve the excitement of sensations that are caused by activation of nerve pathways by trigger points from the sternocleidomastoid muscles. These include the following:

- Reddening of the eye and skin
- Visual disturbance
- Blurring of vision
- Excessive tearing
- Itching and fullness in the ear
- Unilateral deafness
- Tinnitus (but this sound may also be caused by many other things, like working around loud noises and taking too much aspirin or ibuprofen)
- Dizziness

Pain is often felt in the shoulders, in the back of the head, and in the neck muscles. This pain is due to muscle contraction (a condition called myofascial pain dysfunction syndrome).

TMD Treatment

Treatment plans for TMD are as varied as the patients who present with it. Each patient's treatment must be tailored to her or his unique problems and the contributing factors.

Treatment Goals

It is important to realize that the goal of TMD treatment is to minimize pain and restore function. TMD conditions are not "cured," but instead are managed. The basic goal is to allow the muscles and joints to heal through rest and care. Often damage to the joint itself cannot be reversed, but the body can heal it enough to restore function without pain. We also teach you to recognize the symptoms early and to manage them yourself with the tools we give you. This condition can often recur years later, but early care can reduce its severity.

The basic philosophy of treatment is to do the conservative and reversible treatments first. Irreversible treatments, like surgery or orthodontics, are considered only if conservative steps have failed to bring lasting relief. These more radical treatments are rarely used. Most patients respond well to simpler care.

Treatment Modalities

Modes of TMD treatment usually involve oral orthotic appliances, pain medication, or both. In this section we'll look at both and at some additional treatment options.

Oral Orthotics

Night guards, orthotic appliances, or TMJ appliances are designed to protect the teeth from further wear. These also will reduce the severity of grinding at night and allow the muscles to rest. In severe cases, they need to be worn all day as well, to allow the TMJ and muscles to rest.

The intention of providing these devices is to reduce the load on the TM joints and chewing muscle, although some patients report neck-pain relief after wearing the appliance. They are to fit either the upper or lower teeth. We have clinical proof that the upper flat appliances are more effective. Some dentists provide lower appliances, but they should cover the entire lower teeth to prevent the anterior teeth from erupting.

Medication

The medications used for TMD include pain medication, antidepressants, and muscle relaxants. Let's look at each type in turn.

Pain Medication Pain medication can be bought over the counter or prescribed. Often over-the-counter analgesics like ibuprofen are adequate. Sometimes we prescribe medicine similar to ibuprofen but a bit stronger. These medications not only relieve pain, but also reduce inflammation and aid healing. Occasionally a mild muscle relaxant may also be prescribed. Narcotic medications are not very helpful in treating TMD and are rarely prescribed. These and other prescribed medications are usually taken only when pain is severe or at the beginning of TMD treatment. If the pain doesn't subside within a week or two, contact your physician or dentist.

Often, medications are used to simply alleviate symptoms. Yet, there are times when medication, used properly and conservatively, is very beneficial. Various medications are used for different reasons.

Nonsteroidal anti-inflammatory drugs (NSAIDs) help control both pain and inflammation. Over-the-counter NSAIDs include aspirin and ibuprofen. Aspirin is still the drug of choice for pain and inflammation, but ibuprofen (Motrin) is also a good drug for treating these problems.

Acetaminophen (Tylenol) is equally good for pain management, but it doesn't affect inflammation. However, it's kinder to the stomach than aspirin or ibuprofen and is often prescribed for patients with ulcers or stomach problems. Also, aspirin and ibuprofen, taken for a long time, can produce ringing in the ears and bleeding problems. Long-term use of acetaminophen is not without problems, however; it can cause kidney damage. Therefore, none of these medications should be taken for a long time without monitoring by your doctor.

Antidepressants Antidepressants, used in low doses at bedtime, seem to reduce the effect of some brain chemicals that stimulate the body, producing bruxism (grinding or clenching the teeth) and interfering with sleep.

Muscle Relaxants In addition to pain medication, skeletal muscle relaxants, such as Parafon Forte DSC (Chlorzoxazone) may be prescribed. If you take this drug and develop fever, rash, nausea or vomiting, fatigue, dark urine, or yellowing of the skin or the conjunctiva (white part of the eye), notify your doctor immediately. It is also a good idea to avoid drinking alcohol while using this medication.

I have found that Flexeril (Cyclobenzaprine) at bedtime is very effective in reducing muscle pain. In severe cases, for about 4 weeks, I prescribe Skelaxin Metaxalone during the daytime. It's another good muscle relaxant, and doesn't cause drowsiness.

Additional Treatment Options

Jaw Rest You must rest your jaw for it to heal. An occlusal splint will help during sleep but other steps should be taken. Don't chew gum, bite your nails, clench your teeth, or continue any other nonfunctional jaw habits (like pencil chewing and so forth). Your diet should be fairly soft, so avoid chewy and crunchy foods during treatment. When you notice that you're clenching your teeth, relax the muscles by dropping the jaw with your lips together and teeth apart.

Moist Heat Moist heat soothes the sore muscles of TMD. It promotes blood flow into the muscle, which aids in healing and relaxing the muscle. This increased blood flow also helps increase the intake of analgesic/anti-inflammatory medications into the muscles. A wet washcloth with a hot water bottle will do, or you can purchase moist heating pads. Note, however, that for TM joint pain, sometimes an ice pack helps.

Physical Therapy Physical therapy can help to strengthen the muscles, increase joint flexibility, and reduce inflammation. The dentist treating TMJ dysfunctions can provide some simple stretching therapy in the office. A referral to an outside physical therapy facility is highly recommended, but make sure that the facility has personnel well trained to treat TMJ disorders.

Stretches Muscle spasms can sometimes be released by gentle stretching. A good time to do stretching is in the warm, moist environment of the shower or bath, particularly in the morning and before bedtime. Some of these stretches are very simple to perform. Speak to your dentist or physical therapist about a stretching program.

Stress Management Emotion and stress play an important role in TMD. TMD may be a sign that the patient is under stress. Anything that relieves stress is helpful, such as reading, exercising, listening to music, and the like. If the stress is getting to be a bit much, counseling may help you learn how to manage it. It is almost impossible to get relief from TMD if the underlying emotional issues are not addressed. Biofeedback is often used to gradually learn how to reduce muscle contractions.

Referral You may need a specialist to optimally treat your TMD. You can seek opinions and treatment from physicians, oral surgeons, orthodontists, psychotherapists, physical therapists, or prosthodontists. Severe cases may be immediately referred to a pain center or a dentist who focuses on treating temporomandibular disorders.

Self-Management

Keep in mind that, for most people, discomfort from TMD eventually goes away whether treated or not. Simple self-care practices are often effective in easing the symptoms. If you need more treatment, aim for treatment that is conservative and reversible. If possible, avoid treatments that make permanent changes in the bite or jaw.

Here are some tips:

- Avoid chewing gum and clenching your teeth.
- Eat soft foods.
- Eat small bites of food and control yawns to avoid opening your mouth wide.
- Maintain good posture and eat nutritious foods to promote joint and muscle healing.
- Hold the telephone, instead of cradling it against your shoulder.
- Eliminate spasms and pain by administering occlusal appliances, moist heat, and medicines.
- Get counseling, stress reduction, or biofeedback/relaxation training.
- Have misalignment of your teeth corrected and, in severe cases, consider surgery.

If irreversible treatments are recommended, be sure to get a reliable second opinion. Many practitioners, especially dentists, are familiar with the conservative treatment of TMD. Because TMD is usually painful, pain clinics in hospitals and universities are also a good source of advice and second opinions. Specially trained facial-pain experts can often be helpful in diagnosing and treating TMD.

Finding a Specialist

Finding a TMD specialist may be harder than finding another good physician or dentist. Some physicians doubt that TMD exists. Some dentists don't want to deal with TMD and don't listen to their patients' complaints. Ask about the care provider's education, about whether they have any interest in TMD and facial pain, and about any special education and training they have in TMD—including where and how long this training was. Dental schools now exist that have special programs to teach about the management of temporomandibular disorders and orofacial pain. Ask the specialist whether he or she believes in conservative, reversible treatment of the TM joints.

If you're told about braces or surgery or full dental or occlusal adjustments, you should think twice before you start the treatment. The most common treatment methods today are non-invasive and follow the protocol I have described.

Good luck!

References

1. Badley EM, Rasooly I, Webster GK. Relative importance of musculoskeletal disorders as a cause of chronic health problems, disability and health care utilization: findings from the 1990 Ontario Health Survey. *J Rheumatology*. 1994;21:505-514.
2. Anderson HI, Ejlerstsson G, Rosenberg C. Chronic pain in a geographically defined general population: studies of differences in age, gender, social, class and pain localization. *Clin J Pain*. 1993;9:174-182.
3. Kaspo GA. Primary Fibromyalgia syndrome in TMD patients. Based on a clinical study conducted on approximately 460 patients presented to the Center for TMJ Disorders and Orofacial Pain Management; 1994 Poster Clinics, Chicago IL, AAOP Annual Meeting.
4. Shankland WE. *TMJ—its many faces: diagnosis of TMJ and related disorders*. 2nd ed. Columbus, OH: Anadem Publishing; 1996.
5. Okeson J, ed. Orofacial pain: guidelines for assessment, diagnosis, and management. Chicago, IL: Quintessence Pub Co; 1996.

CHAPTER

9

Irritable Bowel Syndrome (IBS) Concurrent with Fibromyalgia

Olafur S. Palsson, PsyD

Donald Moss, PhD

Irritable bowel syndrome (IBS) is a gastrointestinal disorder present in 33–77% of individuals with fibromyalgia.[1] This prevalence rate is far higher than the 10–15% rate of IBS in the general population.[2] This chapter reviews the nature, impact, and treatment of IBS. It also discusses the efforts researchers are making to understand the causes and implications of the surprisingly frequent coexistence of IBS and fibromyalgia in the same individuals.

The Nature of IBS

The diagnosis of IBS is based on a specific cluster of bowel symptoms, primarily recurrent or persistent abdominal pain associated with diarrhea, constipation, or both. Secondary symptoms, such as bloating or the sudden urge to defecate, are also associated with the disorder. Such "supportive symptoms" give doctors more confidence in the diagnosis. A committee of international experts has set criteria (called the "Rome criteria") for the type and frequency of bowel symptoms that warrant a definite diagnosis of IBS.

IBS is one of several "functional" gastrointestinal disorders. A functional disorder is one in which no structural abnormality can be found, but function is disturbed. Therefore, a confident diagnosis generally requires a careful medical evaluation. Sometimes medical tests, such as blood tests or endoscopy, are also needed to rule out biological problems that could account for the symptoms.

Demographics

Epidemiological studies throughout the world indicate that IBS is at least twice as common in women as in men. This gender difference is even more pronounced in medical clinics in the United States, where 75–80% of patients visiting doctors because of IBS are women.[3] The reasons for the predominance of women with the disorder are largely unknown, but various physiological, psychological, social, and cultural explanations have been proposed.[4]

Causes of IBS

The causes of IBS aren't completely understood; however, there is growing recognition among experts that many causal factors are involved and that different factors may cause and maintain IBS in different patients.[5]

In recent years, the most studied causal factor (which is thought by many to play a central role in explaining why IBS symptoms occur) is heightened sensitivity to pain in the intestines. Studies that use pressure generated by a balloon inflated inside the gut suggest that approximately two thirds of IBS patients have abnormally low thresholds for experiencing pain in their bowels.[6] Efforts at developing better drug treatments for IBS often focus on chemical methods to reduce this gut sensitivity.

Research has also shown that the muscles of the intestines are over-reactive in many IBS patients, contracting excessively in response to stimuli like food, stress, and pressure.[7] This is the likely cause of the crampy bowel discomfort many IBS patients feel after meals and under stress.

Over the past several years, it has become clear that dysfunctions in the brain and nervous system play some role in IBS. Studies that take snapshots of activity in the brain, using methods such as positron emission tomography and functional magnetic resonance imaging, show that IBS patients tend to process signals from the bowels in different brain centers than other people. In IBS patients, interpretation of sensations from the bowels appears to occur more in brain centers that handle emotional and threatening information, leading to more distress and suffering from these gut sensations.[8] Abnormalities in the body's processing of serotonin, an important neurotransmitter (i.e., a chemical that helps carry information from one nerve cell to another) in the nerves of the gastrointestinal tract, are partly responsible for IBS symptoms as well.[9] Therefore, several drugs already used for IBS and several under development work by correcting the serotonin transmission system. The functioning of the autonomic nervous system (ANS)—the part of the nervous system that automatically regulates the activity of the internal organs—is often altered in IBS patients.[10] But it has been hard for researchers to detect a consistent pattern of abnormality.

Moreover, in recent years it has become clear that gastrointestinal infection can predispose people to developing IBS. About 25–32% of patients who get bacterial gastroenteritis (often due to food poisoning) develop IBS for the first time afterwards.[11] This postinfectious IBS persists for many years.[12]

Psychological and social factors also play a significant role in IBS symptoms. But unlike the physical factors described above, these factors appear to aggravate, rather than cause, the symptoms. Compared with other medical patients or healthy individuals, IBS patients are more likely to have significant symptoms of depression and anxiety,[13] high levels of stress, and a history of trauma, such as childhood abuse. Having these problems appears to worsen the bowel symptoms, make them less responsive to treatment, and increase the need for medical care.[14]

The Impact of IBS

IBS isn't life-threatening. Many patients fear that having IBS is dangerous or will lead to dangerous medical problems like colon cancer or inflammatory bowel disease (which sometimes causes symptoms similar to IBS but is unlike IBS in that it is characterized by ulcers in the bowel wall). However, there is no evidence that having IBS harms the body or endangers the sufferer. Nonetheless, it is a costly and difficult problem, both for patients and for society. On the average, IBS increases a person's annual health care expenses by 49%.[15] In the United States, the disorder consumes more than $20 billion a year in direct and indirect health care costs.[16]

Many IBS patients have mild symptoms and do not seek medical care. However, the disorder is a significant problem for the minority of patients who have severe symptoms. In addition to the suffering that the symptoms bring, they often leave the patient unable to travel, work outside the home, or participate in social events. And many report that the symptoms substantially undermine intimate relationships with their romantic partners or spouses. Such serious effects of IBS have traditionally been largely unrecognized by both medical professionals and the general public. This is partly because the disorder is so private that people in the patient's social circle are often unaware that he or she suffers from it. It's partly also because the disorder poses no threat of physical harm and is therefore too easily regarded as less serious than many other medical conditions.

Studies in the last 5 years have documented the negative impact of IBS on patients. This knowledge is helping medical professionals see that the patient's well-being must be seriously considered in clinical care. For example, a recent study by Miller and colleagues in England found through a confidential survey that 38% of IBS patients in gastroenterology clinics had contemplated suicide because of their symptoms and their hopelessness about their bowel condition improving.[17] Gralnek and his co-workers reported that some aspects of health-related quality of life are worse for individuals with IBS than for patients with major potentially life-threatening medical disorders, such as diabetes mellitus or even dialysis-dependent end-stage renal disease.[18]

IBS and Fibromyalgia

Scientific study of IBS now examines its overlap with other medical conditions. Researchers have discovered that IBS not only co-occurs at high rates with some other digestive tract disorders, such as functional dyspepsia (stomach distress and indigestion), but also co-occurs at much higher rates than expected with four chronic health problems that have little to do with the intestinal tract: fibromyalgia, chronic fatigue syndrome, temporomandibular joint disorder (TMJ or TMD), and chronic pelvic pain. Of these four, the high rate of co-occurrence between IBS and fibromyalgia is by far the best established. Six studies show that fibromyalgia occurs in 20–65% of IBS patients.[1,19] Conversely, 13 studies report that between 35% and 77% of fibromyalgia patients have IBS. In other words, in samples of patients with either condition, the other occurs at rates so far above normal that this cannot be happening by chance. The reasons for this high overlap are currently a matter of considerable interest to experts.

Common Characteristics of IBS and Fibromyalgia

IBS and fibromyalgia are both chronic and complex conditions that have a number of characteristics in common, as the reader may already have appreciated. Many investigators have examined such commonalities to see if they provide a causal link explaining why these disorders occur together so frequently. Yet it's probably fair to say that, to date, these attempts have resulted in more frustration and confusion than insight. For example, abnormalities in autonomic nervous system function have been repeatedly found in both IBS and fibromyalgia, but the pattern of dysfunction is different and, in some ways, tends in opposite directions in the two disorders.

Stress plays a definite role in both disorders, and hormones involved in the body's response to stress (such as corticotropin-releasing hormone [CRH] and adrenocorticotropin hormone [ACTH]) also show some abnormality in both conditions. But the pattern seems to be exaggerated stress hormone activity in IBS and suppressed activity in fibromyalgia. Pain sensitivity is a shared and central characteristic of both IBS and fibromyalgia, but here again the pattern isn't comparable. In IBS, pain sensitivity is typically increased inside the intestine, but patients don't show the tender points that characterize fibromyalgia. Conversely, when fibromyalgia patients are tested for pain, they show musculoskeletal tenderness but none of the heightened intestinal sensitivity seen in IBS.

And so the physiological patterns of these disorders are proving more different than alike. This fact challenges the view of some medical theorists that fibromyalgia and IBS, along with other chronic health problems, are merely different surface reflections of the same broader "somatic syndrome," with the same underlying physical and psychological causes. Wessely and colleagues[20], who principally promoted this view, had even suggested that which diagnosis patients receive might be happenstance, depending on what kind of medical expert they visit. (For example, in the same patient a rheumatologist might see fibromyalgia and a gastroenterologist might see IBS.) This view seems unwarranted considering the mounting evidence of multiple physiological differences between IBS and fibromyalgia.

The Consequences of Living with Both Disorders

What are the consequences of having *both* IBS and fibromyalgia? A few studies have investigated this question, but the results are inconsistent and make it hard to draw many general conclusions.

One relatively large Italian study recently found that if IBS patients also have fibromyalgia, their bowel symptoms are more severe, but they don't have worse psychological symptoms.[21] An Israeli research team reports that patients who have both IBS and fibromyalgia have poorer quality of life, poorer physical functioning, greater sleep disturbance, and (in contrast with the Italian findings) more psychological distress than those with only one disorder.[22]

They also tested for fibromyalgia tender points in the IBS patients and found that even IBS patients without fibromyalgia had more tender points than people with neither disorder.

Yet Chang and colleagues conducted two smaller studies in the United States that contradicted the Italian findings. They found that IBS patients with fibromyalgia had less abdominal pain than patients suffering only from IBS,[23] and that IBS patients without fibromyalgia were less sensitive to pain at traditional fibromyalgia tender points than even healthy subjects.[24]

Although it is hard to draw firm general conclusions from these data, it seems that having both disorders at least worsens overall physical functioning and quality of life.

Treatment of IBS

As the previous discussion shows, IBS is a mysterious and complicated disorder, and its symptoms appear to result from several variables that may be different from one patient to the next. This makes conventional medical treatment, which typically addresses health problems through focused targeting of a main cause, difficult and relatively ineffective.

In fact, despite the marvels of modern pharmaceuticals and medical technologies, the most frequently used treatment approaches aren't biomedical. The first large-scale survey of medical care for IBS in the United States, conducted in a large health maintenance organization (HMO) in the Seattle area and published in 2004, found that the three most common interventions physicians used were education, reassurance, and suggestions for diet change, such as fiber-rich foods or fiber supplements.[25] These simple methods are often sufficient to help patients with mild IBS symptoms.

For patients with moderate symptoms, one or more of many medications are also used. They treat the most distressing symptoms, such as diarrhea or pain. Such treatments can ameliorate a distressing symptom, but there's little evidence that most of these medications are effective in treating IBS.[26] In the last few years, the first two medications approved for IBS treatment, alosetron and tegaserod, have become available in the United States. However, these drugs are applicable only to certain subsets of patients. Objectively examined, the research shows that few patients benefit more by taking them than by taking any other medication. In controlled research studies, only 5–17% more patients report improvement with them than with a placebo (i.e., with an inert or "fake" pill).[27]

In addition to prescription medications, many IBS patients take over-the-counter medications for their symptoms. Many also use herbal medications and other alternative therapies.

Data on the outcomes of the medical care given IBS patients make it hard to escape the conclusion that it is ineffective. Less than half of IBS patients say they are satisfied with the outcome of conventional medical treatment.[28] The large HMO survey of IBS care by Whitehead and colleagues[25] mentioned above found that 6 months after visiting doctors for their bowel symptoms, only 49% of patients reported being any better and only 22% showed 50% or greater improvement. For patients with the most severe symptoms the rates of improvement were even poorer.

Additional Treatments

The symptoms of patients with severe IBS continue unabated despite their seeing doctors and receiving typical medical care. So, various alternatives or additions to conventional treatment have been, and continue to be, tested. Two such options for severe IBS patients unresponsive to regular medical interventions seem most promising.

One is the use of antidepressant medications. They are often effective in reducing pain even when the patient isn't depressed. (The same has been observed for fibromyalgia.) The older class of antidepressants, called tricyclics, seems more effective than the newer and more popular selective serotonin reuptake inhibitors (SSRIs).

The other effective way to improve outcomes in severe IBS cases is through psychological treatments. A wide range of psychological treatments has been tested, but cognitive-behavioral therapy and hypnosis are currently the two types best supported by research as effective in a large proportion of patients. Both have been shown to reduce the severity of bowel symptoms by 50% or better in some studies,[29] and the benefits often last for years.

The Future Direction of Treatment

We have every reason to believe that IBS treatment will soon become more effective. Several medications are under development, some of which are likely to be more effective than the two currently available. Psychological treatment and antidepressants are becoming more widespread as adjunctive treatments. Furthermore, there is growing interest in testing the benefits of using different treatments in combination, which may be more effective than any particular treatment alone. Finally, treatment will probably become increasingly customized, and therefore more successful, by basing it on tests that identify the causal factors present in each patient.

Much remains to be understood about IBS and how it can be reliably treated. A great deal of research and money is currently devoted to improving our understanding and therapies. And the pace of discovery is accelerating like never before. Getting a better handle on the nature of this complex disorder will also reveal the reasons for the high coincidence of IBS and fibromyalgia, which today continues to be a mystery despite much hard work by researchers.

References

1. Whitehead WE, Palsson O, Jones KR. Systematic review of the comorbidity of irritable bowel syndrome with other disorders: what are the causes and implications? *Gastroenterology.* 2002;122:1140-1156.
2. Drossman DA, Camilleri M, Mayer EA, Whitehead WE. AGA technical review on irritable bowel syndrome. *Gastroenterology.* 2002;123:2108-2131.
3. Russo MW, Gaynes BN, Drossman DA. A national survey of practice patterns of gastroenterologists with comparison to the past two decades. *Journal of Clinical Gastroenterology.* 1999;29:339-343.
4. Heitkemper MM, Jarrett M, Bond EF, Chang L. Impact of sex and gender on irritable bowel syndrome. *Biological Research for Nursing.* 2003;5(1):56-65.
5. Palsson OS, Drossman DA. Psychiatric and psychological dysfunction in irritable bowel syndrome and the role of psychological treatments. *Gastroenterology Clinics of North America.* 2005;34(2):281-303.

6. Whitehead WE, Palsson OS. Is rectal pain sensitivity a biological marker for irritable bowel syndrome: psychological influences on pain perception. *Gastroenterology.* 1998;115:1263-1271.

7. Posserud I, Ersryd A, Simren M. Functional findings in irritable bowel syndrome. *World Journal of Gastroenterology.* 2006;12(18):2830-2838.

8. Ringel Y. Brain research in functional gastrointestinal disorders. *Journal of Clinical Gastroenterology.* 2002;35(Supplement 1):S23-S25.

9. Crowell MD. Role of serotonin in the pathophysiology of the irritable bowel syndrome. *British Journal of Pharmacology.* 2004;141(8):1285-1293.

10. Wood JD. Neuropathophysiology of irritable bowel syndrome. *Journal of Clinical Gastroenterology.* 2002;35(Supplement 1):S11-S22.

11. Rhodes DY, Wallace M. Post-infectious irritable bowel syndrome. *Current Gastroenterology Reports.* 2006;8(4):327-332.

12. Neal KR, Barker L, Spiller RC. Prognosis in post-infective irritable bowel syndrome: a six year follow up study. *Gut.* 2002;51(3):410-413.

13. Palsson OS, Whitehead WE. Comorbidity associated with irritable bowel syndrome. *Psychiatric Annals.* 2005;35(4):320-329.

14. Drossman DA. Do psychosocial factors define symptom severity and patient status in irritable bowel syndrome? *American Journal of Medicine.* 1999;107(5A):41S-50S.

15. Levy RL, Von Korff M, Whitehead WE, Stang P, Saunders K, Jhingran P, et al. Costs of care for irritable bowel syndrome patients in a health maintenance organization. *American Journal of Gastroenterology.* 2001;96:3122-3129.

16. Sandler RS, Everhart JE, Donowitz M, Adams E, Cronin K, Goodman C, et al. The burden of selected digestive diseases in the United States. *Gastroenterology.* 2002;122:1500-1511.

17. Miller V, Hopkins L, Whorwell PJ. Suicidal ideation in patients with irritable bowel syndrome. *Clinical Gastroenterology and Hepatology.* 2004;2(12):1064-1068.

18. Gralnek IM, Hays RD, Kilbourne A, Naliboff B, Mayer EA. The impact of irritable bowel syndrome on health-related quality of life. *Gastroenterology.* 2000;119(3):654-660.

19. Lubrano E, Iovino P, Tremolaterra F, Parsons WJ, Ciacci C, Mazzacca G. Fibromyalgia in patients with irritable bowel syndrome. An association with the severity of the intestinal disorder. *International Journal of Colorectal Diseases.* 2001;16(4):211-215.

20. Wessely S, Nimnuan C, Sharpe M. Functional somatic syndromes: one or many? *Lancet.* 1999;354(9182):936-939.

21. Lubrano E, Iovino P, Tremolaterra F, Parsons WJ, Ciacci C, Mazzacca G. Fibromyalgia in patients with irritable bowel syndrome. An association with the severity of the intestinal disorder. *International Journal of Colorectal Disease.* 2001;16(4):211-215.

22. Sperber AD, Atzmon Y, Neumann L, Weisberg I, Shalit Y, Abu-Shakrah M, Fich A, et al. Fibromyalgia in the irritable bowel syndrome: studies of prevalence and clinical implications. *American Journal of Gastroenterology.* 1999;94(12):3541-3546.

23. Chang L, Berman S, Mayer EA, Suyenobu B, Derbyshire S, Naliboff B, et al. Brain responses to visceral and somatic stimuli in patients with irritable bowel syndrome with and without fibromyalgia. *American Journal of Gastroenterology.* 2003;98(6):1354-1361.

24. Chang L, Mayer EA, Johnson T, FitzGerald LZ, Naliboff B. Differences in somatic perception in female patients with irritable bowel syndrome with and without fibromyalgia. *Pain.* 2000;84(2-3):297-307.

25. Whitehead WE, Levy RL, Von Korff MV, Feld AD, Palsson OS, Turner MJ, et al. Usual medical care for irritable bowel syndrome. *Alimentary Pharmacology 5 Therapeutics.* 2004;20m:1305-1315.

26. American College of Gastroenterology Functional Gastrointestinal Disorders Task Force. Evidence-based position statement on the management of irritable bowel syndrome in North America. *American Journal of Gastroenterology.* 2002;97:S1-S5.

27. Talley NJ. Evaluation of drug treatment in irritable bowel syndrome. *British Journal of Clinical Pharmacolology.* 2003;56(4):362-369.

28. Thompson WG, Heaton KW, Smyth GT, Smyth C. Irritable bowel syndrome: the view from general practice. *European Journal of Gastroenterology & Hepatology.* 1997;9:689-692.

29. Gonsalkorale WM, Houghton LA, Whorwell PJ. Hypnotherapy in irritable bowel syndrome: a large-scale audit of a clinical service with examination of factors influencing responsiveness. *American Journal of Gastroenterology.* 2002;97(4):954-961.

Acupuncture in the Management of Fibromyalgia

Mitch Elkiss, D.O.

Acupuncture is the ancient Indochinese therapy of inserting needles into the body at particular points to relieve pain or other illness. These acupuncture points were discovered both by accident and by trial and error over many centuries. Most lie in particular acutracts, or meridians. Today the acupuncture needles may be warmed or connected to electrodes that deliver tiny electrical stimuli. The goal of acupressure ranges from simple relief of pain symptoms to reversal of an imbalance causing symptoms.

The Ancient Theory of Acupuncture

Traditionally, Eastern medicine views disease as being caused by two types of influences—external and internal. External influences are heat, cold, dryness, dampness, and wind. Internal influences include thoughts, feelings, and so forth. Eastern theory also teaches that we each have three treasures: *Qi* (energy), *Jing* (life essence), and *Shen* (spirit), which represent the vital fluids that circulate along with blood in the acupuncture meridians. These meridians are created by energetic radiations from the deep organs to the body's surface. The acupuncture meridians flow from one to the next in a continuous and well-defined circuit.

Illness, trauma, degeneration, and imbalance block the flow of energy radiations, which causes congestion, fullness behind the blockage, and pain. Downstream from the blockage there is the absence of energy flow. The goal of acupuncture therapy is to help eradicate the blockage, restore normal energy flow, return the system to balance, and alleviate symptoms such as pain, fatigue, and the like.

Modern Theories of Acupuncture

Modern theories suggest that acupuncture stimulates nerve cells, thereby causing them to release more neurotransmitters. Neurotransmitters are chemicals that are used by nerves to communicate with each other. Acupuncture can stimulate nerve cells to release more neurotransmitters, which stimulates energy radiation/electrochemical current flow through the meridians to the brain, spinal cord, and other nerve cell masses. Releasing the blockage in the radiations results in the lessening of pain.

Other current theories invoke the unique properties of the acupoints, their close relation to neurovascular and lymphatic clusters, and their unique relations to the associated connective tissues that serve as an organizational matrix for the body. Recent research suggests that acupuncture affects the brain, causing changes in activity that can be measured on positron emission tomography (PET) scans and functional magnetic resonance imaging (fMRI).[1]

The French Energetic School combines the ancient traditions with the modern discoveries, using the binary logic of yin and yang to explain both sets of observations. It reflects a system of information encryption that reveals imbalances in the body. This system is a tool for instruction, as well as a method of diagnosis and formulating treatment.

Chronic Pain

Pain is one of the great remaining mysteries of medical science. But we are getting ever closer to the answers. We do know that many sets of nerve-cell fibers are involved, each secreting their own neurotransmitter to communicate with the nerve cells they connect to. Some of these neurotransmitters make it easier for the pain-sensing nerve fibers to fire, which increases our sensitivity to pain. Other neurotransmitters make it harder for the nerve fibers to fire, thus decreasing our sensitivity to pain. In other words, some act as an accelerator, and others act as a brake. Morphine, for example, is of the latter type. It kills pain because it *is* a neurotransmitter that inhibits the transmission of pain stimuli. The brain naturally produces it when we are in pain—though not in the massive amounts that a physician can prescribe.

Normally, the brain increases production of opiates and other pain-killing neurotransmitters to desensitize us to pain that doesn't go away.

Chronic pain represents a hyperactive state of the central (brain and spinal cord) and peripheral nervous systems (outside the brain and spinal cord) in which both systems become sensitized to pain. Over time, the nervous systems begin to over-respond to pain stimuli. This means that it takes less stimulation to cause pain and that pain is felt for a much longer period of time following the stimulus.

Moreover, in chronic pain the sympathetic nervous system is often in a heightened state of arousal. The sympathetic nervous system is a massive network of nerves throughout the brain, spinal cord, and body that causes the familiar "fight-or-flight" response, in which the body is almost instantly prepared for a dangerous emergency. Heart rate increases, breathing rate increases, blood pressure rises, emotions flare, adrenalin flows. Needless to stay, it's unhealthy to be in this aroused state more or less permanently. It leads to high blood pressure, irritable bowel symptoms, anxiety, and despair.

Acupuncture for Chronic Pain/Fibromyalgia

In French energetic terms, acupuncture can help reveal and define the energetic imbalance that underlies your symptoms. This helps us understand the path that led to illness and that will lead back to wellness. Understanding the dynamics of becoming unbalanced (i.e., ill) allows us to know what treatment can address both the root (cause) and the branches (symptoms) of your illness. In the traditional Chinese medical (TCM) approach, recognizing a pattern of dysfunction reveals the appropriate intervention. The diagnosis comes from questioning, listening, hearing, palpating points and pulses, and looking at the tongue, facial color, and the sparkle in the eye or lack thereof. In all these systems, the treatment improves circulation of *Qi*, blood, and fluids. Treatment also helps the body's mechanisms for maintaining a steady state, thus moving you toward better balance and better health.

Acupuncture acts on pain-sensing nerve fiber transmission in two ways. One way is by increasing the strength of inhibitory (pain blocking) circuits in the brainstem. The brainstem circuits at the top of the spinal cord act as pain gates that are closed by acupuncture. The other way is by reducing the excitability of pain circuits in the spinal cord and brain. These acupuncture-induced alterations reduce the hypersensitivity of the nervous system that develops in chronic pain. It also works by calming the chronically hyper-aroused sympathetic nervous system, which reduces the muscle contractions present in fibromyalgia.

In all these systems, the treatment improves circulation of *Qi*, blood, and fluids. Treatment also helps the body's mechanisms for maintaining a steady state, thus moving you toward better balance and better health.

How Does Acupuncture Work?

The agent of acupuncture is the needle. Through its bimetallic effects, thermoelectric effects, and electron transfer, it creates a trickle of electrons at the punctured points. This current of tiny injury affects the body's electromagnetic field. We can manipulate the needle to tonify and stimulate or to disperse and sedate.

The body's electromagnetic system allows static electricity at the surface to communicate with its greatest depths. We think electromagnetic information travels in an electro-ionic milieu to its targets through the body's

- Interstices (the spaces between body cells)
- Fascial planes (sheaths around muscles)
- Perineural networks (sheaths around bundles of nerve fibers)
- Cellular microtubular systems (tubes within body cells)

Some of this current is directed through the peripheral nervous system, particularly through the small fibers. Nerve fibers stimulated in the periphery, spinal cord, brainstem, and brain can inhibit pain by increasing inhibitory pain activity and decreasing excitatory pain activity. Even pain modulation mediated by the brain and brainstem is affected by acupuncture.

Because nerves communicate with one another through neurotransmitters, it is logical to conclude that neurotransmitters are involved. For example, endorphins are neurotransmitters that kill pain. Research has shown that acupuncture has a pain-killing effect through increasing the amount of endorphin nerve cells release, especially when stimulated electrically at low frequencies (2–10 Hertz).[2] In fact, it appears that different stimulation frequencies differently affect many neurotransmitters involved in pain, including dynorphins, enkephalins, serotonin, norepinephrine, gamma-aminobutyric acid, and others.

Fibromyalgia

Fibromyalgia is a chronic pain syndrome. Its dominant features are musculoskeletal pain, fatigue, and tender points clustered around the shoulder and hip. There is a host of associated symptoms, chief among them being a nonrestorative sleep pattern. Other symptoms include headache, cognitive impairment, depression, anxiety, irritable bowel syndrome, interstitial cystitis, vulvadynia, premenstrual syndrome, paresthesias, muscle twitching and cramping, dizziness, poor coordination, and sensitivity to chemicals, odors, lights, noises, and medications. Yet there are no physical signs of disease except for the tender points, although electroencephalography has shown alpha waves intruding into the delta wave stages of sleep.

Current thinking understands fibromyalgia as a state of central nervous system hypersensitivity. This could help explain the panorama of possible symptoms associated with fibromyalgia. It can also explain the cutaneous allodynia (pain from a stimulus that normally isn't painful) and hyperpathia (abnormally severe pain from a stimulus that normally is slightly painful).

An Acupuncture Treatment

An acupuncture treatment begins with getting your history and performing a physical examination. Then we formulate a treatment strategy and begin treatment.

Most traditional acupuncture practitioners take thorough histories. Often they ask questions that might seem unusual. They ask about your favorite colors, preferred flavors or those most avoided, and your preferred climates and seasons. They ask questions about your emotional tone. They get a complete medical history of you and your family.

Meanwhile, the practitioner is performing part of the physical examination, observing the quality of your voice and demeanor. They will ask to see your tongue, noting its shape, color, morphology, and coating or lack thereof. Some practitioners try to detect the subtle facial colorations that differentiate the elements (red, yellow, white, black, or green). The idea is to recognize the pattern of disharmony in the patient by identifying which is dominant, which is in excess, and which is deficient.

We also palpate the body, paying attention to tender points and their location. The traditional acupuncture points are palpated to test for tenderness, fullness, or emptiness. We examine the 12 radial pulses that correspond to the 12 acutracts or meridians. We try to discern any difference in the pulses on the right and left side that provide clues about the associated organ and its functioning. Although there are many pulse qualities to look for, they can be roughly characterized as full or not full, fast or slow, slippery or wiry, or even choppy.

For the treatment itself, usually, you wear a gown or loose clothing that permits access to the skin. You take a comfortable position on your back, stomach, side, or, rarely, sitting upright. So you can lie relaxed for 12–20 minutes without moving, we provide pillows and cushions.

Then we insert needles using sterile technique. Typically, we use 12–20 needles. Patients often feel a brief, deep, achy, or numb sensation when we insert a needle. We then leave you to relax quietly with the needles in place. Usually, we dim the lights and cover you lightly to keep you warm.

Sometimes we use needles warmed with burning moxa or mugwort. (Mugwort/moxa is the common name for the plant Artemisia vulgarum. It is dried, burned and used in sticks, cones, and clumps to heat acupuncture points and/or needles in acupuncture points. There are properties to the herb itself above and beyond the heat that it generates.) Other times the needles are clipped to wires attached to electrical stimulators. These stimulators deliver electrical impulses of varied frequency and amplitude to stimulate the needles. Patients typically experience this electrical stimulation as comforting. Sometimes the needles are manipulated gently by hand.

We insert acupuncture needles at these trigger points (shown in Figure 10.1) and often at some acupoints along the spine. After treatment we remove the needles and advise you to refrain from heavy activity, heavy meals, or excitement for 2 or 3 hours.

Usually, we also prescribe some physical exercise. Occasionally we recommend some form of manual therapy or dietary changes. We may also offer advice and treatment aimed at improving sleep quality and cultivating a positive self-image, one capable of feeling better. Sometimes this involves relaxation exercise, meditation, breathing exercise, or guided visual imagery.

Advantages of Acupuncture

Acupuncture has some advantages over traditional Western therapies. For one thing, there are no side effects to speak of from acupuncture. There can be minor bruising and local irritation, but serious side effects are rare. The most serious potential side effect is

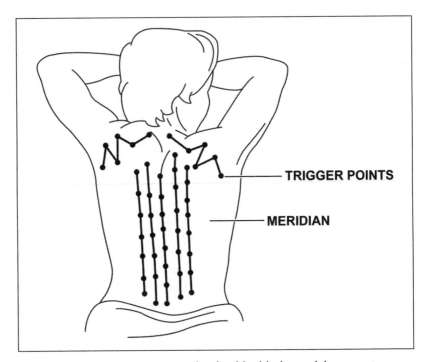

FIGURE 10.1   Trigger points on the shoulder blades and the acupoints along the spine.

organ puncture, but that should never happen. In contrast, all medications have side effects.

At different points in their recovery, many fibromyalgia patients feel pain when pressure is put on trigger points. In fact, people with fibromyalgia often do not tolerate physical therapy or muscle manipulation therapies because they are painful. But with acupuncture the amount of local tissue trauma is minimized, and the needle insertion points are at a distance from the actual tender points.

I have observed beneficial effects from acupuncture in patients suffering with fibromyalgia. These patients report less pain, less use of pain medication, and more stamina. Sometimes the benefits are most notable as a more restorative sleep pattern. Often, after acupuncture, patients report higher energy levels and lower anxiety levels. Even if their pain remains, these benefits improve their quality of life. This may be partly due to the constitutional effects of acupuncture—normalizing effects on a wide range of body functions.

Dietary advice, psychological counsel, individual exercise plans, and recommendations to optimize sleep complete the treatment plan. It seeks to identify imbalance in the system and restore harmony. The acupuncture needle is the tool whose proper placement encourages a new equilibrium for the individual. Acupuncture is a safe tool for treating fibromyalgia patients. Its effectiveness is substantiated by scientific, traditional, and anecdotal reports. This ancient practice represents the medicine of the future.[3]

References

1. Cho ZH. Presentation at American Academy of Medical Acupuncture. 2002.
2. Mussat M. *Physiological Energetics of Acupuncture*. Serejski E, trans. Paris, France: Librairie Le Francois; 1997.
3. Stux G, Pomeranz B. *Acupuncture: textbook and atlas*. Berlin, Germany: Springer-Verlag; 1989.

Visual Problems Concurrent with Fibromyalgia

Randy Houdek, OD

If you have fibromyalgia or chronic fatigue syndrome, visual problems aren't your primary concern. In fact, they aren't a normal consequence of fibromyalgia or chronic fatigue syndrome. But they can arise as bothersome secondary problems that need special attention. These complications fall into two categories:[1]

- Those directly related to the stress and fatigue of the syndromes
- Those that are secondary complications of the various treatment options

In this chapter, I'll explain these two types of problems and what you can do about them. But before we dive in, take a moment to look at Figure 11.1, so you know what I'm talking about when I mention the parts of the eye.

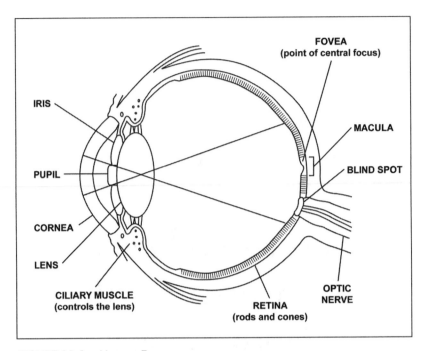

FIGURE 11.1 Human Eye

As you'll see, the eye works much like a camera. It captures an image of what you see and transmits this image through nerve cells to the brain. The brain controls the eyes much like a computer controls data—by sending impulses through wires (nerve cells) that move and focus the eyes.

Now let's look at visual complications directly related to fibromyalgia and chronic fatigue syndrome.

Eye Problems Directly Related to Fibromyalgia

- Dry eye disease (DED)
- Accommodative spasm
- Binocular dysfunction

Let's look further into each of these.

Dry Eye Disease

Although no studies confirm a relationship between dry eye disease (DED) and fibromyalgia or chronic fatigue, many patients with these diseases experience dry-eye symptoms. DED seems to be these patients' most frequent ocular or visual complaint.

In its simplest form, DED is a condition in which the clear front surface of the eye, the cornea, no longer remains moist. Two problems arise. One is that, as the cornea dries, its tissue becomes unhealthy and cloudy. The result is poor, uncorrectable vision. The other problem is discomfort as the eye becomes irritated.

Signs and symptoms of DED can vary in their severity and include foreign body sensation, burning eyes, crusty eyelashes, red and swollen eyelids, blurry vision, fluctuating vision, no tearing, and excessive tearing. Yes, excessive tearing can be a sign of DED; it's an over-reaction to dryness as the normal tear film is quickly depleted. However, it does nothing to correct the underlying problem (refer to Figures 11.2 & 11.3).

The tear film has three layers. The outermost layer is a thin oil layer. This layer prevents the watery tear from evaporating too quickly. The central layer, the thickest, is the aqueous, or watery, layer. This layer provides moisture, nutrients, and oxygen to the cornea. The innermost layer is the mucin layer. It's sticky and "glues" the water layer to the front surface of the cornea. A thinning of any layer can cause DED, which reduces the quantity or quality of the tear.

Many possible causes of DED have been proposed, and they are similar to the proposed causes of fibromyalgia and chronic fatigue syndrome. They include, but are not limited to, autoimmune disease, nervous or motor neural system deficiencies, nutritional deficiencies, hormonal changes, injuries, or surgical intervention.

Dry Eyes Disease Treatment

We now have many options to treat DED, options not only to treat the symptoms, but also to treat the underlying causes. All of the treatments discussed in the following sections should be used under the care of an eye-care professional who monitors their effectiveness and side effects, adjusting treatment accordingly.

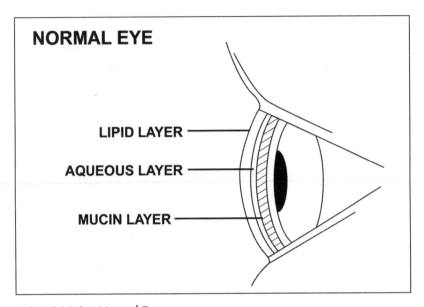

FIGURE 11.2   Normal Eye

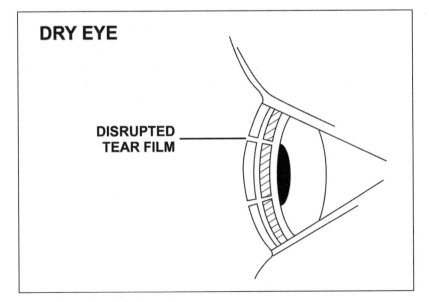

FIGURE 11.3   Dry Eye

Artificial Tears Artificial tears are usually the first line of treatment. There are countless over-the-counter (OTC) formulations on the market. They vary in consistency: some have the consistency of water, some are emulsions, some are gels, and some are ointments. Dosing can be from hourly to once a day. Ointments usually are used for severe conditions, and usually are applied at bedtime. They consist of lanolin and white petroleum jelly, which coat the cornea and blur the vision.

Many eye drops contain preservatives that may cause dryness or may complicate an already compromised cornea, so I recommend that you use formulas without preservatives. Two common preservatives to avoid are benzalkonium chloride and thimerosal. Both can irritate or be toxic to a compromised cornea. Not all preservatives are bad though. Some newer OTC drops contain preservatives that are derivatives of hydrogen peroxide. They are well tolerated and have very low toxicity levels.

There are also nutritional and homeopathic formulations of artificial tears that work very well. Some contain the vitamins A, C, B_6, and B_{12} and the nutritionals bilberry and bee pollen. Some of these are OTC whereas others, though nonprescription, must be purchased through an eye care professional.[2]

Restasis Restasis (cyclosporine, Allergan), is the newest treatment option in the area of drops. It was approved in the United States in December 2002 as a prescription-only drop for the treatment of aqueous deficiency dry eye. Numerous studies show it is effective in treating DED by increasing tear production. Recent reports showing that it also reduces inflammation have made it a more popular option among eye care professionals. A major convenience is that it needs to be used only twice a day.[2]

Ocular Nonsteroidal Anti-inflammatory Drugs (NSAIDs) Eye Drops or Steroid Eye Drops NSAIDs and steroids are used to reduce the pain and inflammation of DED. They are prescription-only medications usually used as a quick fix for severe problems, because they have unwanted side effects like cataract, glaucoma, corneal toxicity, corneal melt, and increased risk of viral infections. Long-term use, for more than even a few months, may be necessary though, so NSAID use must be closely monitored.

Bandage Contact Lenses (BCL) Bandage contact lenses can be used with drops when drops alone do not provide relief. BCLs provide a protective covering for a compromised cornea. You can wear these lenses continuously for up to 30 days. They are especially effective in preventing drying at night due to incomplete lid closure (secondary to muscle fatigue).

Punctal Plugs Punctal plugs are inserts for the canaliculi (tear drainage ducts) to reduce or stop the outflow of the natural tear. By plugging these ducts, punctal plugs allow tears to accumulate before being lost to evaporation. Some are one- to two-week dissolvable plugs of collagen, some are one- to three-month dissolvable ones, and some are semi-permanent inserts of silicone and latex. The last are considered semi-permanent because they can be removed if necessary. Usually, one- to two-week dissolvable plugs are tried first to see if blocking tear drainage helps. If it does, more permanent plugs are inserted. Tear ducts can be permanently blocked by cauterizing them with heat or a laser.

Oral Tetracyclines and Doxycycline Oral tetracyclines and doxycycline are antibiotics that treat lid disease, which can be secondary to stress. We also use them to thin the tear layer oils (refer to Figure 11.3), allowing the tear to better cover the corneal surface. Like all antibiotics, you can take them only for a limited time, so they are but a temporary solution.

Oral Nutritionals Oral nutritionals are vitamins, minerals, and herbs proven effective in treating DED. Like artificial tears, they include vitamins A, C, B_6, and B_{12}; the minerals zinc and selenium; and the omega 3 fatty acids (O3FA). They offset the effects of stress and fatigue to improve the health and metabolism of the cornea and eyelids. Of particular interest are the O3FA. They improve the performance of the meibomian glands (oil glands) in the eyelids, thereby preventing tear evaporation. Some foods high in O3FA are cold-water fish (like salmon, cod, and mackerel), anchovies, sardines, flax seed, and grape seed. We usually recommend that you supplement your diet with 2,000 milligrams daily of fish oil, cod liver oil, flax seed extract, or grape seed extract.[3]

On the Horizon

New treatments for DED will include:

- Secretagogues, which stimulate the secretion of essential tear components
- Mucomimetics, which mimic the mucin layer of the tear film
- Anti-evaporates, which stimulate the oil layer to prevent evaporation[4,5]

Accommodative Spasm

Accommodation is the act of focusing, adjusting the visual system for the distance of what we're looking at, so that the eye always produces a clear image. The process is analogous to focusing a camera. When taking a picture, you use your hand to adjust the lens for a clear image. Likewise, when looking at something, the brain uses eye muscles (ciliary muscles) to adjust the shape of the eye and its lens.

The eye creates an image of what you see on a "screen" at the back called the retina. Nerves in the retina transmit this image to the visual cortex of the brain. The brain analyzes the image and sends commands back to the eye's ciliary muscle, adjusting the focus. The closer an object is to your eye, the greater the adjustment needed and the harder the ciliary muscle must work.

A spasm or inefficiency in this system causes blurry vision, which is the second most common visual complaint of patients with fibromyalgia or chronic fatigue syndrome.

Yet with age, everyone experiences a decrease in the ability to focus. That's because age thickens the eye's lens, reducing its flexibility and the room it has for adjusting. The ciliary muscle, however, still functions. This condition is called presbyopia, and usually begins affecting people around age 40.

Weakness of the ciliary muscle controlling the lens mimics presbyopia. People with fibromyalgia or chronic fatigue syndrome experience this weakness, and it can occur at any age.

The signs and symptoms of a focusing deficit are:

• Blurred near vision
• Headaches with prolonged near work
• Drowsiness
• Decreased interest in reading and other near-point visual activity
• Delayed ability to clear the vision when looking from near to far objects and vice versa

Accommodative Spasm Treatment

To treat focusing problems, eye-care professionals use spectacles, contact lenses, and visual therapy, or a combination of treatments.

Spectacle Lenses Spectacle lenses compensate for, but do not cure, the eye's inability to maintain a clear image on the retina. They may be reading glasses (either full size or half eyes), bifocals, trifocals, or progressive lenses. Full reading glasses make all near objects within a limited range very clear, but objects beyond the focal point look blurry. The other options offer multiple focal points more suited to everyday use, as when looking from a book to the television set.

Contact Lenses Contact lenses work like spectacles. There are many brands of bifocal and multifocal contact lenses, in both the rigid, gas-permeable form and in the soft-lens form. Another option is monovision, in which one eye, usually the dominant one, is corrected for distance vision while the other eye is corrected for near vision.

Visual Therapy Visual therapy exercises the eye to stimulate and increase the flexibility and stamina of the ciliary muscle and its nerve pathway to the brain. It also makes you more aware of visual blur and how to compensate for it. You may need in-office treatments 30–60 minutes long, one or two days a week. It may take from one to six months, or even longer, to accomplish the full treatment. We also give home-based treatment to help fully compensate for the deficit.

Binocular Dysfunction

Binocular dysfunction (BD) is the inability to use the two eyes together efficiently. Although BD isn't as common as DED or accommodative spasm, this problem is very visually disturbing.

Six muscles per eye control eye movement. So, 12 muscles must work in unison to maintain single binocular vision. General malaise or fatigue in any one of them reduces the efficiency in coordination of these muscles, causing visual disturbances. These disturbances include diplopia (double vision), dizziness, nausea, reduction in depth perception, words running together, re-reading sentences, and fatigue with near work.

Binocular Dysfunction Treatment

Treatment options include lenses, prisms, patching, and visual therapy. Treatment for BD can be difficult though, because dysfunction can vary from day to day depending on the individual's health.

Lenses Depending on the degree of dysfunction, lenses (such as bifocals and progressive lenses) similar to those used for accommodative spasms may help. You may need several pairs, however, to meet specific needs at specific distances.

Prisms Prisms are similar to lenses, but instead of compensating for a focusing blur, they re-align the eyes to compensate for a double-image blur. Prisms are harder to prescribe than lenses. The prescription specifies not only their power, but also a direction, because double vision may be horizontal, vertical, or oblique. BD can vary with the malaise, so there are prisms that you can apply to, and remove from, your spectacle lenses like plastic window stickers. You can cut them into any shape to fit any spectacle frame.

Patching Patching, or blocking, vision in one eye is yet another option. We use it only when the two eyes cannot be comfortably re-aligned with any other method and double vision remains. Be aware that when an eye is patched, the entire visual field of that eye is eliminated. As a result, you lose depth perception. Therefore, when wearing a patch, you must be cautious, especially when driving, walking, or using the stairs. Hopefully, you would need a patch infrequently and for short periods only.

Visual Therapy Visual therapy similar to that used for accommodative spasm can significantly help BD. It improves the quality of vision, thereby reducing visual fatigue and the dizziness and nausea that may accompany BD.

Complications Secondary to Treatment Options

The side effects of oral medications that are used to treat fibromyalgia/ chronic fatigue syndrome can cause complications, although most of them are temporary and reversible. These side effects don't just occur with prescription medications; they can also occur with over-the-counter medications. In the following sections I list a few common medications and their potential side effects. Notice that dry eye disease, accommodative spasms, and binocular dysfunction are among these side effects. Also note that conjunctivitis (pink eye) is usually an allergic reaction and therefore not contagious.[3]

Analgesics (Painkillers)

Acetaminophen (Tylenol) can cause reduced color vision, conjunctivitis (allergic), and decreased vision.

Aspirin can cause reduced color vision, conjunctivitis, decreased vision, DED, and a transient increase in nearsightedness (reduced distance vision with improved near vision).

Narcotics including propoxyphene napsylate (Darvocet), Oxycodone HCl (Oxycontin), and Tramadol HCl (Ultram) can cause eye problems. Darvocet can cause hallucinations and visual disturbances, Oxycontin can cause miosis (small pinpoint pupils), and Ultram can cause hallucinations and cataracts.[7]

NSAIDs

Ibuprofen (Motrin and Advil) can cause blurred and/or reduced vision, scotomata (blind spots), binocular dysfunction, and reduced color vision. Naproxen (Anaprox and Aleve) can cause visual disturbances.[7]

Corticosteroids (Anti-Inflammatory)

Corticosteroids are steroids that have an anti-inflammatory effect. They include prednisone and dexamethasone (Decadron). In general, all oral corticosteroids increase the risk of nonreversible posterior subcapsular cataracts, glaucoma, and viral and fungal eye infections.[7]

Antidepressants

Antidepressants include Elavil, Fluoxetine HCl (Prozac), and Sertraline HCl (Zoloft). Elavil can cause mydriasis (large pupils) and cycloplegia (accommodative spasm/paralysis). Prozac can cause blurred vision, DED, mydriasis, double vision (binocular dysfunction), ptosis (droopy eyelid), and conjunctivitis. Zoloft can cause eye pain, accommodative spasms, and conjunctivitis.[7]

Muscle Relaxants

Muscle relaxants that can be problematic include cyclobenzaprine (Flexeril), carisoprodol (Soma), and methocarbamol (Robaxin). Generally, these medications produce the most varied side effects: mydriasis, blurry vision, accommodative spasm, binocular dysfunction, increased risk of narrow-angle glaucoma, visual hallucinations, and retinal hemorrhages (bleeding in the back of the eye).[7]

Anti-Anxiety

Anti-anxiety medications include alprazolam (Xanax), clonazepam (Klonopin), and lorazepam (Ativan). These drugs are benzodiazepines that can cause decreased corneal reflex, conjunctivitis, accommodative spasm resulting in blurry vision, and binocular dysfunction leading to double vision and decreased depth perception.[7]

Anti-Seizure

Anti-seizure medications include carbamazepine (Tegretol) and gabapentin (Neurontin). They can cause binocular dysfunction with double vision, nystagmus (involuntary shaking of the eyes leading to reduced vision), DED, photophobia (light sensitivity), and visual field defects.[7]

These are just a sampling of medications used to help relieve the symptoms of fibromyalgia and chronic fatigue syndrome. The number of potential side effects seems great, but remember that they are dose dependent, infrequent, and usually reversible when the medication is withdrawn. *Always let your primary physician know if any unusual signs or symptoms occur.*

Considering all the aches, pains, and fatigue you have with fibromyalgia and chronic fatigue syndrome, the eye problems seem minor. But, when they occur, they may seem worse than they are, because our sense of sight, the process of vision, and the eye's comfort are highly energy dependent. Fortunately, there are many treatments to reduce your discomfort and rectify the abnormalities.

References

1. Fibromyalgia Treatment. proHealth ImmuneSupport.com. Available at: http://immunesupport.com/fibromyalgia-treatment.htm. Accessed March 1, 2007.
2. Karpecki PM. Dry eye treatment. *Review of Optometry.*   Available at: http://revoptom.com/index.asp?page=2_1483.htm. Accessed March 1, 2007.
3. Nichols KK. Nutraceuticals and dry eyes. *Contact Lens Spectrum.* June 2005.
4. Murphy J. Dry eye: signs vs. symptoms. *Review of Optometry.* June 2004: 53-61. Available at: http://revoptom.com/index.asp?page=2_1483.htm. Accessed March 1, 2007.
5. Byrne J. Investigational dry eye drugs address the disease on several levels. *Primary Care Optometry News.* November 2005:16.
6. Fraunfelder FW, Fraunfelder FT. Ocular toxicology. *Clinical Ophthalmology.* Vol. 5. Chapter 37.
7. Pellegrino M. ImmuneSupport.com. Treatment & Research Information, *Prescribed Medications for Fibromyalgia.* 2002.

12

Coming to Terms with Chronic Pain

Peter Ianni, PhD

Your behavior affects fibromyalgia pain. This chapter outlines how you can modify your behavior patterns to reduce the pain and retain the ability to do more with fewer pain flares. These techniques mitigate the effects of fibromyalgia on the nervous system. To understand them, you need to understand how the nervous system is affected by fibromyalgia.

Fibromyalgia and the Nervous System

We know that fibromyalgia affects the nervous system. Specifically, it affects the central nervous system and the autonomic nervous system. The central nervous system is the brain and spinal cord. The autonomic nervous system is a system of nerve fibers in the brain, spinal cord, and throughout the body that automatically controls life processes by regulating things like heart rate, blood pressure, sweating, digestive processes, body temperature, various reflexes, and so forth.

The autonomic nervous system has two divisions, one that works like an accelerator and one that works like a brake. These divisions, or subsystems, are called the sympathetic nervous system and the parasympathetic nervous system. Generally, the sympathetic nervous system serves as the accelerator, stimulating activity, and the parasympathetic nervous system serves as the brake, inhibiting or slowing activity.

In fibromyalgia, nerve fibers in the central nervous system[1] and the *sympathetic* division[2] of the autonomic nervous system become more sensitive and more active than normal. In fact, evidence suggests that the higher incidence of fibromyalgia in females is due to sex-linked differences in autonomic and central nervous system responsivity.

A general firing of nerves throughout the sympathetic nervous system causes what is known as the "fight-or-flight" response. It is triggered by trauma, fear, anger, or cold and prepares us to react physically and emotionally to emergencies. Many changes occur throughout the body in this state:

- Heart rate increases.
- Blood vessels to most organs and the extremities constrict to maintain core temperature.
- Our mood is greatly affected.
- Many other changes occur that make us better able to cope with danger and injury.

In an emergency, these reactions of the sympathetic nervous system can be life-saving, but this hyper-aroused state should be temporary, or it will have bad effects on the body. Unfortunately, chronic activation of the sympathetic nervous system also occurs when people are in a great deal of pain.

Fibromyalgia patients suffer from chronic excessive sympathetic activation. One effect is cold hands and feet due to constriction of blood vessels in the fingers and toes. Research shows that this constriction is greater in females than males.[3] This suggests that the sympathetic fight-or-flight response has a greater effect in females and explains the higher rate of fibromyalgia in females. In any case, more females than males suffer from Raynaud's disease, a disorder that causes painful coldness and color changes in the fingers and toes. Many people with fibromyalgia also suffer from Raynaud's attacks.

In addition, when pain signals travel to the brain they stimulate several structures in it, including the amygdala, the anger center.[4] Anger is a hard-wired response to pain, and it stimulates the sympathetic nervous system.

Some argue that sympathetic nerve activation is the primary cause of fibromyalgia pain[2] because the sympathetic nervous system includes both (1) fibers that transmit pain signals from the body to the brain and (2) fibers that transmit contraction signals from the brain to the muscles. When muscles contract, they compress blood vessels so that tissues don't get enough oxygen, and that can cause pain.

One research group[5] developed an animal model showing that any intense pain causes muscles in the painful area to contract, a response known as the *withdrawal reflex*. For example, menstrual cramps can trigger withdrawal reflexes in women. So can whiplash, burns, fractures, and disc/joint degeneration.

Because pain causes anger, anger stimulates the sympathetic nervous system, and the sympathetic nervous system can cause pain, a vicious cycle can commence. Normally, however, that doesn't happen. Normally, the brain habituates (gets used to) repetitive pain signals and becomes less sensitive to them. This has a natural pain-killing effect.

But the brains of fibromyalgia patients do not habituate properly. The thalamus is a filtering structure in the brain that filters out repetitive pain signals, but it is underactive in fibromyalgia patients.[6] Drugs known as serotonin reuptake inhibitors reduce chronic pain by increasing thalamic filtering.[7]

In addition, pain activates many more brain *areas* in fibromyalgia patients than in other people—a phenomenon known as *central sensitization*.[8]

Both central sensitization and the failure to habituate amplify pain and other sensations (e.g., cold, heat, touch, odors, and smoke) that can be painful when amplified. This condition is known as allodynia, and it occurs in many patients with intractable pain.[9]

Thus, excessive autonomic and central nervous system activation occurs in chronic pain. The result is not only increased pain, but also decreased cognitive functioning. Figure 12.1 shows the relationship between central and sympathetic nervous system activation and cognitive functioning.

Cognition is the mental process of knowing, and includes such things as thinking, reasoning, remembering, awareness, and perception. These complex functions take place in the outer layer (cortex) of the brain. In Figure 12.1 you can see that we are most mentally "with it" when we are wide awake but not highly aroused. Hence excessive activation of the cortex and the autonomic nervous system caused by severe pain results in not just more pain, but also memory and concentration difficulties, word-finding difficulties, fatigue, and frustration, among other things.

Treatment

Medications that reduce sympathetic activation peripherally don't help, because they cause low blood pressure (dizziness, fainting) and other unpleasant side effects without reducing pain.[2] Medications that reduce brain activation do help, but they must be carefully

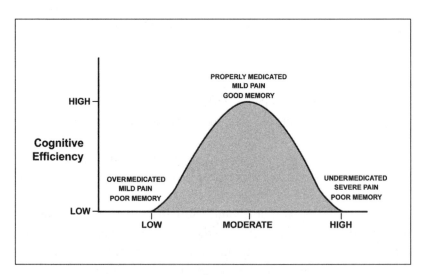

FIGURE 12.1   Autonomic & Central Nervous System Activation[10]

titrated to a dose that achieves pain control without sedative side effects due to overmedication. These include anticonvulsants, selective serotonin reuptake inhibitors (SSRIs), serotonin and norepinephrine reuptake inhibitors (SNRIs), and opioids.[11] Your doctor does not manage your moderate-to-severe fibromyalgia using such medications alone. He or she addresses your symptoms with multidisciplinary, carefully timed interventions to get the best pain control with the least side effects and the highest level of functioning.

You should not rely solely on medication to manage your pain. By adjusting your behavior, you can lessen the pain and minimize the amount of medication you need. The aim is to reduce neurologic activation and pain.

Let's look at some steps you can take to do that.

Some steps are easy and healthy, like wearing sunglasses and avoiding loud noises and bright lights. Some steps are easy but unhealthy, like eating sweets and carbohydrate-rich foods. These foods reduce activation, frustration, and pain,[12] but relying too heavily on them brings unhealthy results. Drinking alcohol to excess temporarily reduces activation and pain but is very unhealthy. Nicotine relaxes muscles and has a mild analgesic effect, but everyone knows how unhealthy smoking is. Taking a lot of sedative medication reduces activation and pain, but you end up drooling on your shoes.

Now for the healthy, more difficult steps you can take. Note that the following recommendations are based on my work with real fibromyalgia patients who have been able to increase their activity levels, have less pain, and feel better.

Emotional Work

Allow yourself to grieve your reduced functional capacities. Each activity you're no longer able to engage in causes a grief reaction. Grief is the feeling of loss, such as in the loss of a loved one. Mourning a loss is a process with five stages[13]:

1. Denial
2. Anger
3. Bargaining with God (when applicable)
4. Sadness/depression
5. Acceptance

Reaching acceptance means that you aren't denying your limitations and you feel less sad and angry.

Feelings of loss develop as fibromyalgia progresses from mild to moderate to severe. Patients with mild fibromyalgia feel little loss, because they can still do things the way they've always done them, even though they have mild pain. For patients with moderate or severe pain, it's a different story. Many are stuck in the anger (resentfulness) or sadness (depression) stages. Some go back and forth between stages. Others accept the loss of some functional capacities but not others, remaining in the denial, anger, bargaining-with-God, or sadness/depression stage about them.

If you are stuck in the denial stage, you don't admit to having functional limitations. You repeatedly exceed your functional limits and then crash (i.e., get stuck in bed for days or go to an emergency room). When you suffer a pain flare, try to identify the cause, which is often overdoing some activity.

When you overwork muscles, tiny fibers in them tear, releasing fluids that can cause severe pain. When you repeatedly overdo, your functional capacities deteriorate. Although you may be getting more done today, you will pay for it later and won't be able to do as much in the long run. Focus on your long-term goal of being able to do more in the future. When you stay within your limits, you have fewer pain flares, you can reduce your medication, and your functional capacities will increase.

Some fibromyalgia patients are stuck in the anger stage. They haven't accepted their reduced functional capacities or their pain. This causes angry feelings, which activate the sympathetic nervous system, reduce thalamic filtering, and increase central sensitization—causing more pain.

To see how this works, let's look at what normally happens to the average person when they get very angry. The average American gets very angry once per week, and they don't fully express the intensity of their anger to the person who hurt them.[14] Afterwards, they think about the event several times during the next few days. Thinking about the event arouses angry feelings, but the feelings about the hurtful person change, as the anger lessens and is resolved. However, when anger isn't resolved in this way, the angry feelings take a long time to subside.

The feelings also take longer to subside when people don't allow themselves to feel their anger at all (denial). Denying anger creates tension (including muscle tension), which remains in the body much longer than a few days. Other people ruminate (intensely reliving/thinking about the event) and remain angry instead of letting the anger subside over a few days. Rumination is a poor way of coping with angry feelings. Denial and rumination are anger management methods that increase pain.

If you find yourself getting very angry more than once per week, work on managing your angry feelings better. It's much more complicated than counting to 10.

If a particular person is triggering angry feelings, he or she may be hurtful, critical, or emotionally abusive. Sometimes a person doesn't mean to be hypercritical, and letting them know they are hurting you is all you need to do. To maintain the integrity of the relationship, they will avoid doing what hurts you. But if this person remains hypercritical or abusive, consider (1) distancing yourself from that person, (2) asking them to participate in some counseling with you, or (3) getting some counseling yourself.

A relationship involves repeated interactions between two people, and both share some responsibility for each other's feelings.

If you have a relationship that needs much repair, remember that everyone wants to feel loved. It isn't enough for *you* to know that you love someone; *they* need to feel loved in your tone and accepting attitude. Too much criticism causes hurt and angry feelings that can wreck a relationship. When you're having a bad pain day, say so. Apologize for hurting others with your crankiness, and learn to be conscious of how your words feel to the other person.

If you are bargaining with God to have the pain taken away, you are heading for trouble. Having a spiritual life helps people cope with pain,[15] but bargaining with God causes resentment when the pain isn't taken away. Ask God for the strength to cope with your pain symptoms.

Some fibromyalgia patients are stuck in the sadness stage. They no longer deny their loss of functional capacity reductions, but their feelings of loss can be overwhelming. Those of us without fibromyalgia know what our functional capacity limitations are, and we accept them. The same is true of people with mild fibromyalgia, because their pain doesn't interfere with how much they can do. But when you become unable to engage in activities that give you a sense of accomplishment, you lose the joy those activities brought you. Absent that joy is great sadness. So, it is important to find new activities that restore that sense of accomplishment without increasing the pain.

Think outside the box: container vegetable/herb gardening, talking to support group co-members, listening to talking books, cooking for scout groups, volunteering, and so on. If the sadness becomes overwhelming and you feel hopeless, talk to someone you trust (a minister or health professional) about what you should do.

As you get through the emotional work needed to resolve your feelings of loss, you can get to work figuring out what pain management techniques work for you. These may include some of the following.

Behavioral Pain Management Techniques

Certain activities can reduce sympathetic and central nervous system activation. Play quiet, calming music; avoid noisy environments; wear ear plugs; dress warmly in cold temperatures; shop when stores aren't crowded; avoid loud nasty people; soak in a hot tub or whirlpool; use heating pads; and so forth.

Slow down. Hurrying activates the sympathetic nervous system.[16] It causes your muscles to contract more. Understand that slowing down is hard to do. Initially, your psyche will rebel, because it associates hurrying with goal achievement. *The faster I go, the more tasks I can complete per unit time. When I slow down, I feel like I'm not getting anything done.* Slowing down is hard, because it reduces short-term feelings of accomplishment. This can arouse feelings of inadequacy, laziness, and guilt.

Learn to conserve. If you have moderate to severe fibromyalgia and you want to attend a wedding on Saturday, get plenty of rest on Thursday and Friday. Get your clothing ready several days in advance. On the day of the wedding, get some rest after the ceremony and before the reception. Make sure you have a comfortable chair (bring a pillow if necessary); try to find a comfortable seating position; take breaks in the lounge or sit in your car when you need to. Don't plan much for the next day, so you can give your body a chance to recover.

Prioritize. If you want to give your child the quality time he or she needs, don't try to keep an immaculate house. Your children aren't going to remember that the house was clean. But they may remember that you preferred to do housework than spend time playing with them. The same goes for your mate. When your mate returns from work, he or she may be more pleased if the house is a little messy but you are feeling good, are in a good mood, and can be up and around.

Figure out how to move/position your body without increasing the pain. This may sound easy, but it can be difficult. Severe pain is so traumatizing to the psyche that, once it subsides, the psyche tries to forget how bad it was. Therefore, it's hard to remember what movements you should avoid. In addition, patterns of body movement are overlearned habits that we do automatically. For years, a fellow with severe lower back pain bent at the waist to brush his two dogs every day. One day he tried sitting on a footstool and was amazed at how much less pain he experienced when he brushed his dogs in this new position.

If you catastrophize, learn to stop it. Research shows that when you ruminate about all the terrible things that are going to happen, your brain hyper-activates, amplifying your pain.[17] It is hard to stop catastrophizing, because moderate to severe pain causes a chronically ego-regressed state. This means that your mind functions at a level that it did when you were younger—a time when you were overwhelmed by the challenges facing you. When you have significant ego regression, you may have rapid mood changes and lack self-discipline. Resist the urge to beat yourself up. Again, it is hard to do, but you can do it over time.

Practice mindfulness. Try to enjoy your surroundings (air, plants, people, music, etc.) to their fullest. This requires mental discipline and a refocus on the *quality* of your experiences as opposed to the quantity of them. What we really desire is contentment with what we have, which requires that we stop focusing on what we don't have. It is human nature to take what we have for granted, and it is important to work on not doing so.

Practice deep relaxation techniques. If your pain levels are relatively mild (1, 2, 3 on a scale where 0 = no pain and 10 = amputation without anesthesia), you may be able to relax deeply enough to reduce your pain levels. If your pain is moderate (4, 5, 6/10) or severe (7, 8, 9, 10/10) you probably cannot relax your muscles deeply enough to make a difference. One reason is that severe pain triggers a stronger withdrawal reflex.

But biofeedback training can help you in this situation, so that you learn how to relax muscles and reduce nervous system activation. Your biofeedback therapist should be warm and positive—cold therapists interfere with the training process. During biofeedback training, you learn how to focus on relaxing the body despite the pain. How hard this is depends on pain intensity, proper medication management, involvement in dysfunctional relationships, and your level of acceptance.

Some people prefer to set aside time to practice relaxation techniques, while others find it easier to practice relaxation throughout the day.

When people without intractable pain give you advice on pain management, remember that they are trying to help. They tell you what works for them. They may suggest that you go out for lunch to take your mind off the pain. They may tell you to just ignore the pain or distract yourself. These techniques work very well for people with episodic, everyday[18] mild pain, but they do not work for moderate to severe pain. If you go out to lunch on a bad day, you will wonder why you did this to yourself. You can push through mild pain, and it will subside on its own, but if you push through moderate to severe pain, you will put yourself in agony. Learn to recognize whether the advice applies to you. If it doesn't, graciously explain, if the advice giver seems interested. If the advice giver isn't receptive, accept that and move on.

Cut yourself some slack. When you are in a lot of pain, your memory storage and retrieval functions are compromised. If you're in a lot of pain when someone tells you something, you may not store it properly and, if it hasn't been stored properly, you won't be able to retrieve it at a later date. Even if the information was stored effectively, it won't be retrievable if you're in a lot of pain when trying to remember what you were told. Many other cognitive functions are affected by pain including attention/concentration, problem solving, cognitive flexibility, etc.

Finally, understand that pain results in regression of important ego functions. Ego functions refer to how we respond to challenges from our external and internal environments. As long as you are healthy, you can handle challenges better at age 20 than when you are 10; you can handle challenges better when you are 30 than when you're 20, etc. The complexity and strength of one's ego functions often peaks in our 50's however there is theoretically no age limit to developing our ego functions further.

When you are in severe pain, your ego regresses to an earlier age, usually to your adolescence. You become moody and overwhelmed by everyday challenges like when you were 17, 15, 13 or younger. Ego function regression is real and is experienced to some degree by all who are in the traumatic state caused by severe intractable pain.[19]

If you are in severe pain, understand ego regression and why you are feeling so overwhelmed. Anyone in this much pain would feel this way.

This chapter has outlined the challenges faced by people dealing with mild, moderate and severe pain. Most of the recommendations apply to all types of chronic pain conditions. If you are fortunate to be suffering from only mild pain, the aforementioned suggestions may help you to keep the pain from getting worse. If you suffer from moderate to severe pain, your top priority should be to get the pain under control by learning about your disorder and doing what needs to be done. Fight this battle wisely.

References

1. Yunus MB. The concept of central sensitivity syndromes. In: Wallace DJ, Clauw DJ, eds. *Fibromyalgia and Other Central Pain Syndromes.* Philadelphia, Pa: Lippincott, Williams & Wilkins; 2005:29-44.
2. Martinez-Lavin M. Dysfunction of the autonomic nervous system in chronic pain syndromes. In: Wallace DJ, Clauw DJ, eds. *Fibromyalgia and Other Central Pain Syndromes.* Philadelphia, Pa: Lippincott, Williams & Wilkins; 2005:81-87.
3. Cooke JP, Creager MA, Osmundson PJ, Shepherd JT. Sex differences in control of cutaneous blood flow. *Circulation.* 1990;82:1607-1615.

4. Westlund KN. Neurophysiology of nociception. In: Pappagallo M, ed. *The Neurological Basis of Pain.* New York, NY: McGraw Hill; 2005:3-19.
5. Giambardino MA, Affaitati G, Lerza R, De Laurentis S. Neurophysiological basis of visceral pain. *J Musculoskeletal Pain.* 2002;10:151-163.
6. Graceley RH, Bradley LA. Functional imaging of pain. In: Wallace DJ, Clauw DJ, eds. *Fibromyalgia and Other Central Pain Syndromes.* Philadelphia, Pa: Lippincott, Williams & Wilkins; 2005:89-100.
7. Arnold L. Systemic therapies for chronic pain. In: Wallace DJ, Clauw DJ, eds. *Fibromyalgia and Other Central Pain Syndromes.* Philadelphia, Pa: Lippincott, Williams & Wilkins; 2005:365-388.
8. Gracely RH, Petzke F, Wolf JM, Clauw DJ. Functional MRI evidence of augmented pain processing in fibromyalgia. *Arthritis Rheum.* 2002;46:1333-1343.
9. Hoffer MJ. The neurophysiology of pain. In: Aronoff GM, ed. *Evaluation and Treatment of Chronic Pain.* Baltimore, Md: Williams & Wilkins; 1992:10-25.
10. Yerkes RM, Dodson JD. The relation of strength of stimulus to rapidity of habit formation. *J of Comparative and Neurology and Psychology.* 1908;18:459-482.
11. Coluzzi F, Mattia C. Antidepressants, anticonvulsants and miscellaneous agents. In: Pappagallo M, ed. *The Neurological Basis of Pain.* New York, NY: McGraw Hill; 2005:581-598.
12. Wurtman RJ, Wurtman JJ. Brain serotonin, carbohydrate craving, obesity and depression. *Obesity Research.* 1995;3:477S-480S.
13. Kubler-Ross E. *On Death and Dying.* New York, NY: Simon & Schuster; 1993.
14. Averill J. *Anger and Aggression. An Essay on Emotion.* New York, NY: Springer-Verlag; 1982.
15. Culver MD, Kell MJ. Working with chronic pain patients: spirituality as part of the treatment protocol. *Amer J of Pain Management.* 1995;5:55-61.
16. Surwit RS, Williams RB Jr, Shapiro D. *Behavioral Approaches to Cardiovascular Disease.* New York, NY: Academic Press; 1982.
17. Gracely RH, Geisser ME, Geisecke T, Clauw DJ. Pain catastrophizing and neural responses to pain among persons with fibromyalgia. *Brain.* 2004;127(4):835-843.
18. Sternbach RA. Pain and 'hassles' in the United States: findings of the Nuprin report. *Pain.* 1986;27(1):69-80.
19. Krystal H. Integration & self-healing, affect, trauma alexithymia. Hillsdale: The Analytic Press; 1988.

ADHD and Fibromyalgia: Related Conditions?

Joel L. Young, MD

Judith Redmond, MA

As Gregor Samsa awoke one morning from uneasy dreams, he found himself transformed in his bed . . . . What has happened to me? he thought. It was no dream . . . . Gregor's eyes turned to the window, and the overcast sky—one could hear rain drops beating on the window gutter—made him quite melancholy. What about sleeping a little longer and forgetting all this nonsense, he thought, but it could not be done for he was accustomed to sleep on his right side. . . . he began to feel a dull ache . . . He felt a slight itching up on his belly; . . . he slid down again into his former position. This getting up early, he thought, makes one quite stupid. A man needs his sleep . . . He looked at the alarm clock ticking on the chest . . . It was half-past six o'clock and the hands were quietly moving on, it was even past the half-hour, and it was getting on toward a quarter to seven. Had the alarm clock not gone off? From the bed one could see that it had been properly set . . . Yes, but was it possible to sleep quietly through that ear-splitting noise? Well, he had not slept quietly, yet apparently all the more soundly for that. But what was he to do now? The next train went at seven o'clock; to catch that he would need to hurry like mad . . . "Gregor," said his father now from the left-hand room, "the chief clerk has come and wants to know why you didn't catch the early train. We don't know what to say to him. . . ." "But, sir," cried Gregor, beside himself . . . . "A slight illness, an attack of giddiness, has kept me from getting up. I'm still lying in bed. But I feel all right again. I'm getting out of bed now. Just give me a moment or two longer! I'm not quite so well as I thought."

—*The Metamorphosis* by Franz Kafka (1916)

Franz Kafka's 90-year-old description of Gregor Samsa's plight describes familiar territory to patients suffering from fibromyalgia. Gregor awakens one morning finding that he has changed into a beetle laying helplessly on his back, legs and arms flailing in every direction. He struggles heroically to accomplish what is, for most people, a routine and mundane daily event—the simple act of getting out of bed. Gregor is highly motivated to fulfill his duties; he simply cannot.

Like Gregor, fibromyalgia patients have disabling fatigue, muscle pain, depression, and poor sleep. They suffer from unseen but disabling symptoms that result in employment loss, family disapproval, and sometimes, a personal sense of disgrace. Gregor's plight and suffering are seared into the minds of students of introductory European literature. The fibromyalgia patient endures more anonymously.

Mental health professionals receive little training in fibromyalgia and related conditions. Many times therapists learn about their patient's frustration over their chronic pain and fatigue in psychotherapy. Fibromyalgia sufferers feel marginalized by the health care system, and rightly so; in general physicians believe these patients are malingering or drug seeking. Fibromyalgia patients respond to this perceived rejection by seeking alternative care, ranging from chiropractic to vitamin therapy and naturopathic medicine.

We who write this chapter were no exception. Our exposure to the condition resulted from our primary clinical interests, depression and attention deficit hyperactivity disorder (ADHD) in adults. In our psychiatric center, we have had the opportunity to observe patients with these complaints over the past 15 years. We found a strong relationship between long-standing ADHD and the development of chronic pain conditions. This chapter serves to describe this clinical picture.

Surprising Early Findings

Besides reporting classic ADHD symptoms, many of these patients complained of severe muscle pain, unrelenting fatigue, abdominal distress, and intermittent headaches. A proportion had been previously diagnosed with fibromyalgia syndrome (FMS), chronic fatigue syndrome (CFS), irritable bowel syndrome (IBS), Epstein-Barr syndrome, or Lyme's disease. A substantial number had histories of migraine headache, tinnitus (ringing in the ears), interstitial cystitis (pain in the urogenital system), and restless legs syndrome (RLS). Most were frustrated; they had consulted many clinicians yet found little lasting relief. Patients heard that their symptoms were unusual or "atypical" to use the medical parlance. Most believed that medical doctors dismissed their complaints after several therapeutic failures.

Initially our clinic dutifully recorded the symptoms of pain and fatigue, but did not specifically address them. Instead, we focused on the patient's primary reason for coming to our clinic—complaints of inattention, distractibility, and hyperactivity. Those who were identified as having ADHD were started on standard medications. Surprisingly, many patients reported improvement in both their ADHD and pain symptoms.

These serendipitous findings forced us to explore the connection between ADHD and fibromyalgia. Are they independent conditions with overlapping symptoms or the same condition dissimilarly labeled by doctors of different specialties? Is it possible that a rheumatologist would diagnose fibromyalgia and a psychiatrist evaluating the identical complaints would diagnose ADHD? Does this relationship explain why similar medications ameliorate seemingly disparate symptoms ranging from distractibility to fatigue and from pain to insomnia? Only careful clinical trials will conclusively answer these questions. This chapter endeavors to explain this relationship.

Although fibromyalgia was the most common chronic-pain condition encountered, we enlarged the definition to include many of the above noted chronic pain conditions we found to be associated with ADHD. Throughout this chapter, we will call this condition the ADHD/fibromyalgia and related symptoms complex (AFRSC).

Disease-State Impact

AFRSC patients are common and have a profound clinical and economic impact. Fibromyalgia is the second-most-reported rheumatologic condition, affecting approximately 4–6 million Americans. The Centers for Disease Control estimates that chronic fatigue syndrome affects between 75 and 265 people per 100,000 in the US population. Approximately half a million people in the United States have CFS or a similar condition. More than 8 million Americans have ADHD.[1]

Taken together, these conditions have huge societal costs; they result in worker absenteeism, workplace inefficiency, and decreased income. The 2000 Annual Statistical Report on the Social Security Disability Insurance Program reports that 661,900 workers received disability payments. AFRSC may cost $60 billion annually, much of that accounted for in productivity loss, medical treatment, and direct disability payments. The human price on the individual's self-concept and family relationships are less tangible, but profound. An understanding of the individual clinical conditions that comprise AFRSC is essential.

ADHD

Attention deficit hyperactivity disorder (ADHD) is a neuro-behavioral disorder that affects 3–9% of school-age children. At least 60% of ADHD children have symptoms that persist into adulthood. By the latest estimate, 4.4% of US adults have the condition.[2] ADHD may not have been diagnosed during the patient's youth, but adults who obtain the diagnosis generally can retrospectively piece together childhood symptoms. ADHD is transmitted genetically, from generation to generation, with a high degree of heritability.

ADHD patients have long-standing symptoms of hyperactivity, impulsivity, and inattention. (See Table 13.1.) Although most normal individuals have a smattering of these symptoms, the diagnosis of ADHD is limited to individuals who have the full constellation of symptoms and to those whose symptoms cause impairment in daily life.

ADHD Diagnosis

Making an accurate ADHD diagnosis requires a comprehensive clinical interview that elicits the patient's past and current symptoms.

TABLE 13.1 ADHD: DSM-IV TR Symptoms

Hyperactivity
• Squirms and fidgets
• Runs/climbs excessively
• Can't work quietly
• "On the go"/"Driven by a Motor"
• Talks excessively
Impulsivity
• Blurts out answers
• Can't wait turn
• Intrudes/interrupts others
Inattention
• Careless
• Difficulty sustaining attention in activity
• Doesn't listen
• Doesn't follow through
• Poorly organized
• Avoids and dislikes tasks requiring sustained mental effort
• Loses important items
• Easily distracted
• Forgetful in daily activities

Fortunately, clinicians can screen for the condition quickly and accurately. The Adult ADHD Self-Report Scale (Adult ASRS) is a carefully researched symptom checklist that quantifies symptoms and level of impairments. Patients can complete this screening checklist in five minutes.

In most settings, ADHD in adults is under-diagnosed. Certain features should alert the clinician that ADHD is a diagnostic consideration. The ASRS should be administered to patients who complain of stress-related physical symptoms, particularly if there are few physical findings. It is important to rule out ADHD in patients with a history of alcohol and drug abuse as well as those who have had only a partial response to a trial of antidepressant medications. Having a child or relative with ADHD increases the likelihood of an adult diagnosis.[3]

ADHD presents in three basic variations:

- Predominantly hyperactive/impulsive type
- Predominantly inattentive type
- Combined type

Predominantly hyperactive/impulsive ADHD fits the popularly held notion of ADHD. Behavioral problems and poor school performance are expected. It is more common in youngsters, and in boys more than girls. With age, hyperactive symptoms diminish.

The predominantly inattentive type of ADHD may be devoid of any hyperactive or impulsive features. The hallmark of these patients is their struggle to stay focused and motivated. They daydream and feel easily overwhelmed by stressful events. As they age, they are more likely than their hyperactive brethren to battle anxiety and depression.

The combined type of ADHD is the most common subtype and affects the bulk of afflicted patients. Combined type patients have a wide spectrum of hyperactive, impulsive, and inattentive symptoms. Most patients suffering from the ADHD/fibromyalgia and related symptoms complex (AFRSC) emerge from inattentive or combined types.

ADHD Impact on Health and Relationships

Recent studies reveal much about ADHD impairments. Compared to others, ADHD adults are laid off more frequently and have lower job status. They are more likely to have interpersonal difficulties with employers and fellow workers. ADHD also has a negative impact on health and perhaps life expectancy. ADHD adults are twice as likely to be dependent on nicotine and alcohol. As a group, patients with predominantly hyperactive/impulsive type ADHD are risk takers and sometimes disregard the potential consequences of their behavior. They have a high rate of motor vehicle accidents.[4]

ADHD Myths

Many myths and misconceptions surround ADHD. Although it is more commonly *diagnosed* in boys, girls and women have the condition nearly as often. Many critics assert that ADHD is over-diagnosed. At least in the adult population, the opposite is true. It is estimated that only 2 million of the 9 million adults with ADHD are diagnosed and only half of those are treated. Although ADHD is considered to be a childhood disorder, most children with ADHD will have persistent symptoms throughout their lives. Perhaps the most common misunderstanding is that hyperactivity is an essential symptom for diagnosis. It is not. In fact, most girls and women with ADHD have the inattentive or mixed type. Many women who otherwise meet criteria for ADHD deny that they have ever been hyperactive (although they might have children who are). Many believe that the stimulant medications prescribed are easily abused and misused. In reality, diversion to others and misuse of the prescription occur predominantly with short, not longer acting stimulants.[5]

AFRSC

Our clinic studied the apparent connection between ADHD and fibromyalgia. Over an 18-month period 70 patients who self-reported having fibromyalgia were evaluated by a psychiatrist and rheumatologist. Nearly all believed that they had a rheumatologic illness such as fibromyalgia, chronic fatigue syndrome, or systemic lupus. Forty percent had a previous diagnosis of depression, but only a few identified themselves as having a primary psychiatric condition.

On physical examination, the rheumatologist concluded that only a small number had a true rheumatological condition. Using rating scales and a psychiatric interview, about 80% of this self-referred, self-described fibromyalgia population met criteria for ADHD. This percentage is far higher than would be expected in the general population. Most had inattentive-type or combined-type ADHD. The study was observational only and did not include a medication trial.[6]

A Proposed Linkage

Other researchers have grouped ADHD together with chronic pain syndromes and other psychiatric problems. James I. Hudson and his colleagues describe affective spectrum disorder, which encompasses major depressive disorder, ADHD, fibromyalgia, generalized anxiety disorder, irritable bowel syndrome, chronic migraines, and other anxiety disorders. Hudson theorizes that these disorders are at least partially responsive to antidepressant medications.[7]

In the last few years, the relationship between physical and psychiatric symptoms has gained traction in the treatment community. Duloxetine (Cymbalta), an antidepressant with dual properties of reuptake, joins an older agent, venlafaxine (Effexor XR), as an effective treatment for painful symptoms associated with depression. This class of antidepressant medication affects chemical receptors in both the brain and spinal cord. Although not "pain medications" in the traditional sense, they alter the way the nervous system processes a painful stimulus. Hence duloxetine has proved a rapid and effective treatment for painful diabetic neuropathy even in patients who aren't depressed.[8]

Although the use of dual reuptake inhibitors (serotonin and norepinephrine) prevails throughout the psychiatric community, our clinical experience points to the central role that dopamine-modulating medications (i.e., ADHD medications) play in the treatment of AFRSC. Unfortunately, studies examining the effectiveness of psychostimulants in AFRSC haven't been completed. However, corollary evidence to support this hypothesis is available. This evidence concerns pramipexole (Mirapex), a drug that increases the amount of dopamine in the brain and is used to treat both Parkinson's disease and restless leg syndrome. Pramipexole was also studied in fibromyalgia patients. Compared with a control group, pramipexole-treated patients noted significant improvements in pain, fatigue, and overall functioning.[9]

A Case Study

Helen, a 57-year-old woman, presented for evaluation because of depression and unrelenting fatigue. She reported feeling "tired all my life" but recently felt she was "unable to crawl out of my cave." Helen's youngest children had recently left for college, and she hoped to return to graduate school to obtain a master's of social work and fulfill a lifelong desire. While pursuing her early coursework, Helen fell asleep during reading assignments. "It brings me back to how I felt 30 years ago in college," she said. Despite being academically capable, her attention drifted in class. She missed simple instructions and often had to ask fellow students for class notes and assignment due dates. "It's embarrassing," she said, "I think people feel I am taking advantage of them. It makes me wonder if I have Alzheimer's disease."

Helen struggled at home as well. She routinely misplaced important documents and household bills. Her friends complained that she didn't return phone calls. Helen's three sisters had long debated whether she was rude; they all felt that during conversations she was preoccupied with other thoughts. "Are we not interesting enough?"

Helen had been married to a pharmacist for 26 years. Throughout the marriage, she was so frequently ill with colds and coughs, that he wondered whether she had an immunological deficiency. For the past 10 years, Helen complained of muscle and joint pain. Her husband arranged for a comprehensive evaluation at the regional academic medical center. A rheumatologist concluded that Helen had trigger points and sent her for laboratory studies. All her blood work to check for an underactive thyroid and rheumatoid arthritis lupus was negative. Epstein-Barr titers were not elevated. Fibromyalgia was the final diagnosis.

When multiple pain medications were unsuccessful, Helen consulted a sleep specialist. The specialist initially considered obstructive sleep apnea or possibly narcolepsy, but formal sleep studies and blood work were unremarkable. Despite the negative studies and out of desperation, her doctors started the standard treatment for obstructive apnea, central positive airway pressure—a method of blowing air into her lungs. It too was not helpful. By default, Helen received the diagnosis of chronic fatigue syndrome.

To combat fatigue, Helen had become caffeine-dependent; it was not unusual for her to consume four diet Cokes in a day. Her tendency to fall asleep while driving prevented her from driving long distances. In fact, persistent drowsiness and inattentiveness may have contributed to a recent automobile accident.

Helen's many ongoing complaints taxed her otherwise strong marital relationship, and her exasperated husband insisted that she consult a psychiatrist. The psychiatrist found Helen to have a gentle, self-deprecating sense of humor. She appeared more frustrated than depressed, and was distressed with her inability to perform at a level consistent with her ability and motivation.

The psychiatric examination revealed that Helen had a family history of depression and attention deficit hyperactivity disorder. Both her mother and grandmother were diagnosed with atypical forms of depression, and over the years both received antidepressant medications. Helen's brother never graduated from high school despite excellent aptitude. Her oldest child was very hyperactive and oppositional as a child, and two nephews had been on psycho-stimulant medications since grade school.

Intermittently through the marriage, Helen battled episodes of depression. Five years earlier, her father had died, and for nearly 18 months Helen grieved. During this period, she often slept more than 12 hours per day. Supportive psychotherapy and antidepressant medications elevated her mood, but gave her sexual side effects.

Since her father's death, Helen's doctors kept her on antidepressant medications and successively prescribed sertraline (Zoloft), escitalopram (Lexapro), and duloxetine (Cymbalta). The medications were moderately helpful but did not significantly improve her chronic fatigue. Helen's sleep doctor gave her samples of modafinil (Provigil), a wakefulness promoting medication. This did improve her alertness, but her new managed care plan claimed that, since she did not have narcolepsy, her policy would not cover the medication.

Clinical Assessment and Outcome

Based on her comprehensive psychiatric clinical interview and relying on ADHD rating scales and other standardized metrics, Helen's psychiatrist diagnosed her with ADHD, predominantly-inattentive type.

Treatment

Helen was skeptical of the diagnosis but agreed to start a morning dose of Adderall XR. Within three weeks, she titrated up to 30 mg every morning. One month later she returned to the psychiatrist's office. "I can focus on what the professor is saying, and I am able to stay awake in class." Helen noted that she completed her assignments and submitted them on time. Her note taking improved. Some of her symptoms returned after 3 p.m., so her doctor added an afternoon dose of short-acting Adderall.

At her next monthly visit, Helen reported that this adjustment improved her ability to fall asleep. She reported far more energy, less depression, and significantly enhanced confidence. She excelled in her graduate seminars, and her family complained less frequently about her inattention and irritability. Helen reported as dramatic a reduction of generalized pain. "My muscles are not so tight. I feel less tension in my neck and shoulders." Helen's progress continued the following month. She no longer felt the need to see her chiropractor and reduced her pain medications to once or twice weekly. Over the next several months, Helen stayed on her medication and reported that "all was going well." Her progress was interrupted when she misplaced her prescription while traveling. "Within a few days I hurt as much as I did before treatment. Only then did I fully realize what the medicine did for me." Since then, Helen has remained on treatment.

We Need to Know More

We suggest that among the adult ADHD population, a subgroup develops fibromyalgia, chronic fatigue syndrome, and related conditions like headaches, irritable bowel syndrome, tinnitus, restless leg syndrome, and other chronic pain syndromes. We have referred to this illness as the ADHD/fibromyalgia and related symptoms complex (AFRSC). AFRSC patients obtain various diagnoses including systemic lupus, chronic fatigue syndrome, and rheumatoid arthritis. Office visits to specialists and various treatments may produce little tangible improvement.

It is important to consider that ADHD may be at the core of some of these conditions. ADHD symptoms are evident in childhood and historically predate most patients' pain and fatigue complaints. Our own research shows that, among self-referred fibromyalgia patients, a large number, perhaps 80%, meet criteria for ADHD.

Helen's case study describes a typical response AFRSC patients have to amphetamine-based stimulants. What drives this response? Perhaps stimulants help patients filter an unpleasant stimulus. In other words, perhaps stimulants alter the way the brain processes pain instead of reducing the actual end-organ pain. Using the model of dual reuptake inhibitors, we conceptualize chronic pain and fatigue conditions as central (brain) rather than peripheral (end-organ) processes.

It should not be lost that this proposed linkage is an early hypothesis. Much more research must be done before clinical recommendations can be conclusive. A working theory undergoes a long process before it becomes a clinical practice. If ADHD proves to be a common factor in chronic conditions, primary care physicians, rheumatologists, and other specialists will have to adopt psychotropic medications. There is precedent for this though. Two decades ago, most doctors did not treat clinical depression, but now nonpsychiatrists write more than half of all anti-depressant prescriptions.

Physicians need to be advocates for their patients. Like Gregor Samsa, the people described in this chapter live on the margins of society, and they may suffer for decades. Current treatments are insufficient. Therefore, the relationship of ADHD to other conditions surely deserves greater scrutiny.

References

1. Aaron LA, Burke MM, Buchwald D. Overlapping conditions among patients with chronic fatigue syndrome, fibromyalgia, and temporomandibular disorder. *Arch Intern Med.* 2000;160(2):221-227.

2. Kessler RC. *American Journal of Psychiatry.* 2006;163:716-723.

3. Adler GK, Valdis FM, Creskoff KW. Neuroendocrine abnormalities in fibromyalgia. *Pain and Headache Reports.* 2002;6:289-298.

4. American College of Rheumatology webpage. Fibromyalgia factsheet. Available at: http://www.rheumatology.org/public/factsheets/fibromya_new.asp?aud=pat.

5. American Psychiatric Association. *Diagnostic and Statistical Manual of Mental Disorders.* 4th ed. Washington, DC: American Psychiatric Association; 1994.

6. Arnold LM, Hess EV, Hudson JI, Welge JA, Berno SE, Keck PE Jr. *American Journal of Medicine.* 2002;112(3).

7. Barkley RA. Attention-deficit hyperactivity disorder. *Scientific American.* September 1998;66-71.

8. Barkley RA. *Attention-Deficit Hyperactivity Disorder: A Handbook for Diagnosis and Treatment.* 2nd ed. New York, NY: The Guilford Press; 1996:201-224.

9. Holman AJ, Myers RR. *Treatment of fibromyalgia syndrome with the dopamine3 receptor agonist pramipexole: a double-blinded randomized placebo-controlled trial.* American College of Rheumatology meeting; San Antonio, TX; Oct 16-21, 2004; Abstract L 19.

A Guy's Perspective:
The Other 20% of
the Fibro Population

Robert S. Leider

*Rob is a retired high school principal with a high level of
ability, creativity, and commitment to every endeavor he
undertakes. He is married and has two high school
children. He is an avid reader and freelance writer.*

— •◆• —

I read, I listen, I hear that guys don't get fibromyalgia. Mostly
women get it. But guys do get it, and I got it bad.

If his family and friends don't believe in it—if even his doctors
don't believe in it—a guy who has it is weak. He's lazy. He hasn't "the
stuff" to be a tough man. He's wimpy, a whiner. He can't take it,

can't even win a British game of darts at the pub, let alone be considered for a good brawl old-west or Indiana-Jones style. It keeps him from being a "regular guy."

Most of the time we men just shut up about it—the pains, the aches, the waves of exhaustion—and just behave badly. We get grumpy with our family, friends, and eventually even our co-workers and bosses. This is a male thing akin to not asking for directions or waiting until your leg falls off to drag your butt to a doctor. But even if you have seen the doctor, a great doctor who understands your pain, exhaustion, and clumsiness, the support of the doc alone can't relieve you of the pressure. We men are under pressure to provide for our families, to move heavy objects, to participate in sports, to play ball with our kids—to be who we really are.

The doubts, the fears, and the pains start an emotional and physical downward spiral, and the further down a guy spirals, the more maladaptive he becomes in handling this demon called fibromyalgia. Yelling, cursing, lengthy isolation, self-exclusion. And then finally just passing out cold on the sofa, or, in my case, hiding behind the sofa. "Quality of life" (he says in a sarcastic tone) becomes *work/sofa, work/sofa. Work/sofa, no work/sofa. Sofa, sofa, sofa.* Depression, pain, and more hiding. Hiding from yourself, hiding from the people you love, the people you have always been strong for and found satisfying self-esteem in being strong and capable for, 24/7.

The incessant aches, pains, spasms, and muscle weakness, plus the cloudy thinking begin to take their toll. Your circle of family, friends, and co-workers—most of whom are sympathetic and concerned (if you bothered to tell them you have a problem, which most guys don't)—slowly, surreptitiously, turn away. Until one day, either you have nobody left to project your rotten, whiny attitude on or you finally listen to the best advice someone tried to give you there in the dungeon of your mind: "Go to a doctor."

Finding the right doctor is another story, especially if it is 1986 and you've had an automobile accident that left you with brain injury, broken bones, memory struggles, and the onset of what you'll come to know as post-traumatic fibromyalgia. That guy, the clueless, undirected, wandering-through-each-day guy, was me.

The accident happened in the summer of 1986. A kid who'd had his driver's license for but a week plowed through a red light and a stop sign, taking me out through the driver's door of my Pontiac 1984 6000 woody wagon. The impact sent me flying to the right, and the rebound from the seatbelt sent my head left into the metal between the driver and passenger doors. My legs and arms bashed into the dash and steering wheel (no airbags yet). My glasses flew who-knows-where (though the EMS technicians found them and a couple of teeth). At the hospital I didn't know the answers to all those questions admissions asks you, like Who's the president? What year is it? How old are you?

Two years of cognitive rehab, physical therapy, unexplained pains, and a search for myself dragged by. I knew only what people told me, what I saw in pictures and on paper. Indeed, I knew only that I knew nothing, not even half the people I was supposed to know. Somehow, through the tenacity of my building principal and by doing pretty much what people told me to do, I held down my job two or three days a week as a high school drama teacher. Fortunately, drama teachers can *be* a little screwy. So, I made it through, with the help of my students (whom I called by the names of students I'd taught 10 years earlier), my great friends on the staff, the wonderful substitutes, and the principal, who is one of my personal heroes, because he didn't listen to the therapists or doctors and let me retire a disabled wreck.

In 1989 I married a saint who lived and breathed by the book *The Man Who Mistook His Wife for a Hat*, tolerating with great compassion my odd behaviors and misunderstood physical ills. We had our first child mostly because the good folks at cognitive rehab said I would not mistake the child for a turkey and cook it, and I had come so far along that, despite taking my wallet out of my pants pocket and ceremoniously laying it on the roof of the Jeep (yes, I was driving) every time I got into the car, we could start a normal family.

I was now back to work four days a week, directing plays; advising the yearbook; teaching theatre, speech, and English; and working on our 1928 Tudor home with my power tools—except for the electric screwdriver, which had been taken away from me for my own protection because I was distracted so easily, though I still managed to drill through one of my fingers.

When the brain fog began to clear, I became more aware of nagging pains, physical exhaustion in addition to mental exhaustion, muscles not working, painful deep bumps that radiated pain (trigger points), skin rashes, and areas so sensitive I couldn't even touch them. I was watching someone I didn't know from the outside in, and I didn't care much for that person.

The rehab team recommended a physiatrist they worked with. He told me I wasn't crazy. Do you realize how big that was? I wasn't crazy! Yes, as we knew, the head injury was real, the cognitive challenges were real, *and* the pain was real. Though he called the overall malady "fibromyalgia," he said it was more complicated than usual, because the ailment was either induced by the trauma or allowed to emerge by it.

He started me on a course of pills, patches, and injections in places that blew me away. Injections of maricaine, cortisone, and other potions under my shoulder blades, under the base of my neck—back and front—in my hands, arms, and shoulders. Later he showed me on a chart that these were trigger points. I had, and still have, trigger points as big as golf balls. In fact, I've given them names like "the alien colonies" and "Mr. Big Knot."

Time spent in the waiting room and examination room was never less than three hours, but I went because, for the most part, the treatments helped. Eventually, the physician developed a medical condition that forced his retirement.

Through my physical therapist, I found another doctor, whom many of my former doctor's patients also found and migrated to. He is simply a genius in understanding fibromyalgia and the nervous system. He was so accurate with his injections that I began to get relief for months at a time. He also understood the depths of fibro and how it can eat away at every facet of your life.

I never told anybody I had fibromyalgia. As a guy I still thought it wasn't cool. If anyone asked, I alluded to my car accident, some falls I'd had, scoliosis—but not fibromyalgia. The only people I could share the secret name with were two of our building secretaries who had it. One was my own assistant, and she had it very bad. She says that I was a good boss, because I understood her bad days. We laughed with dark humor at how pathetic we were when we both were having a fibro day. However, if I hadn't had this condition myself, as a manager I wouldn't have had the compassion to understand my co-worker's pain and dilemma.

Through the fall of 2005, I lived with the pain through regular treatments with injections, ice, heat, exercise, and the impossible task of making my A++ personality rest. With medication I managed the depression from the constant pain. And, despite my exhaustion, I kept myself busy right up until bedtime, thus pushing the pain aside to ignore it as best I could, and then knocked myself out for the night with another prescription.

For all this time, I acknowledged my understanding of it to people who said they had "the fibro" as I nicknamed it, but I never told anyone I had it. I didn't even tell my kids, though I did often beg them to press their elbows deeply into Daddy's knots. In fact, I would often catch a football player in the hallway at school and ask them to "push with your elbow, right here, with all your weight." Sure it was probably inappropriate, but again, I was the drama teacher, kooky and well-liked. So, thinking it was pretty funny, I managed to maintain this off-beat survival technique to create more pain in the area of pain, putting the real pain at bay, like when a magician distracts you.

I no longer even discussed the issues with my wife, who at one time was my advisor. She got tired of telling me to take it easy and to quit being so stubborn when it was obvious that I should rest but did yard work anyway—for 4 hours only to crash then for 24 in agony. Other times she knew I would just get crabby, go to the physiatrist, get the shots, come home and lie on ice, take something, and then be pretty normal for a few weeks.

It's funny in an odd way that I could tell one friend another friend tragically had cancer but not talk about fibromyalgia. Why, after all this time? Maybe because few people realize how bad it can be and don't care or understand the disease and its devastating tentacles into your life. Or maybe because it isn't "chi-chi" mainstream enough to be acceptable and good lunch talk? Because it certainly isn't guys-at-the-bar-after-softball talk; I can tell you it ain't.

Am I going to trade my Hawaiian camp shirts for t-shirts blazoned in orange printer's ink with the slogan, "FIBRO BOY" or "Be nice to me, I have fibromyalgia and I hurt all the time!" (It isn't funny, though you've got to laugh to make light of the burden, or it will eventually drag you down and crush you.)

I still seek out the multi-purpose, pointed pieces of wood and therapy canes I use to crush knots—as well as convenient doorknobs, lidocaine patches, ice balls, and any other creative mechanism I can come up with to bring about temporary relief. And I would say I have been fairly successful, until this fall.

I fell down a dozen wooden deck stairs behind my house and took out both feet, both ankles, both legs, and a knee. I crushed a heel and fractured some ribs, some vertebrae, my shoulder, and some cheekbones. It has been a ridiculously long recovery. I have so much metal that I'll never get through an airport again. But the worst part is that *The Fibro* took full advantage of the fall and subsequent surgeries: It has knocked me so far down that, as I reach the end of this chapter, I also reach my last day of work.

The fibro won this round, and I'm retiring at the end of the month. The people around me at work have been encouraging and supportive, but I am beat, exhausted. I hurt like hell, and thank God that I can at least still think and write, even through the plethora of knots and trigger points.

Yes, Mr. Big and the crew are up and running. All you can do is look outside yourself and find the humor, somehow, in the whole mess. The be-a-man training in me says to get movin', and eventually I will. You cannot lie down with this thing and quasi-croak. You must find something you can do. You must do it every day.

As wicked as the fibromyalgia is, it is a devil you can beat.

And maybe eventually some guy friends will even understand it.

CHAPTER
15

Physical Therapy Evaluation and Treatment of Fibromyalgia

Loren DeVinney, PT, OMPT

Physical therapy plays an important role in managing fibromyalgia (FM) syndrome. Like many other diseases and syndromes, fibromyalgia is best treated by a multidisciplinary team coordinated by a medical doctor familiar with FM. Physical therapists are an important part of this team, because they understand pathology (the study of disease) and provide unique techniques.

Most of this chapter is about the physical therapy treatments I have found most effective when working with fibromyalgia patients. First we'll cover the following topics:

- The basic brain and muscle dysfunctional components of fibromyalgia
- The challenges involved in managing pain and dysfunction

Brain and Muscle Dysfunction

Central Nervous System Hypersensitivity

From a physical therapist perspective, central nervous system hypersensitivity means a patient is experiencing too much pain, and we have to block or modify the pain sensations. Fibromyalgia patients' brains don't filter or properly dampen the pain (and other) signals that come from their bodies. Their brains amplify normal and abnormal sensations, leading to the perception of pain. Tight muscles may not be tender in a healthy person, but they can be extremely painful in an FM patient.[1]

Muscle Abnormalities

Fibromyalgic muscles are tender, painful, or both. Research shows structural abnormalities in the muscle fibers, which are primarily due to not enough oxygen (hypoxia). These abnormalities cause pain (refer to Figure 15.1).

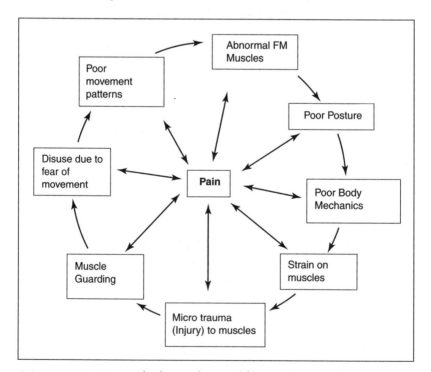

FIGURE 15.1   Pain cycle due to abnormal fibromyalgia muscles

Special Challenges in Managing Fibromyalgia

Some health care practitioners do not understand fibromyalgia, so fibromyalgia patients are often not properly treated. They have much pain and tenderness but many normal diagnostic findings. Standard physical examination tests, such as X-rays or blood tests, are negative.

Another complication is that fibromyalgia is not easily cured. Health professionals can find this frustrating and a threat to their feelings of competence. Many professionals prefer to work with acute pain problems (lasting less than six months) because they feel gratified by the rapid progress they see their patients making. Fibromyalgia patients are chronic patients (i.e., their pain problems are probably going to last longer than six months).

Developing a Treatment Plan

Before beginning treatment, a physical therapist examines the patient. That examination consists of two parts:

1. The first part is largely subjective. The therapist reviews your medical history and listens to your account of your current problems, including any pain and loss of function.
2. The second part is largely objective. The therapist performs a physical examination, tests, and measurements.

Then the PT assesses, or evaluates, the findings. This assessment is our professional interpretation of both the subjective and objective findings in the examination.

Finally, we develop a treatment plan.

The Examination

First the physical therapist examines the patient. The exam consists of two parts:

3. The therapist reviews your medical history and asks about your current problems, including pain and loss of function.
4. The therapist then performs a physical examination, tests, and measurements.

The Subjective History

Fibromyalgia patients most often report a long history of pain, with or without a specific injury. They are experiencing pain in many areas, typically on both sides of the upper and lower body. Other medical problems, such as irritable bowel syndrome or poor sleep, are common. Frequently we find that the patient reports depression or appears depressed.

Typical Objective Findings

Objective findings are things the physical therapist observes and measures with standard reproducible tests. In other words, if another therapist performed the same tests on the patient, the findings would be nearly identical.

Specific, multiple areas of tenderness are, of course, considered the main diagnostic feature of FM. But tenderness is fairly subjective. Palpating patients' muscles and counting the number of tender/trigger points in the 18 recognized places provides a number that can be compared as treatment progresses or flare-ups occur.

Fibromyalgia patients' muscles have a unique texture and feel. Their soft tissue (which includes skin, muscle, fascia, and tendon) feels different from that of patients who have other injuries or other problems. Normal soft tissue has a soft, pliable texture. Fibromyalgia patients' have thicker, stiff tissue that is best described as having a "gunky" feel to it. Even after their pain is better, their flexibility improves, and their trigger points subside, their muscles still feel "gunky".

Other objective findings may include the following:

- Poor posture
- Impaired gait (i.e., a limp or pain in walking)
- Altered range of motion and movement (e.g., the patient is unable to turn his or her head far enough to look behind)
- Strength/endurance deficits
- Widespread tenderness

Finally, the subjective and objective findings are reviewed with the patient and a plan of care determined.

Plan of Care

We discuss both short- and long-term goals with the patient, as well as the best course of action to achieve these goals. With the patient's input, we construct a plan of care that includes specific treatments and the expected frequency and duration of these treatments.

Physical Therapy Treatments

We address the central hypersensitivity by blocking or calming the pain. Heat, cold, and ultrasound calm the pain signals, and electrical stimulation can block the signals. Manual therapy to release peripheral nerve and myofascial tissue can reduce the abnormal pain signals, reducing central sensitivity. It is important for the therapist to know when to apply myofascial release, when to strengthen, and when to begin aerobic exercise.

Fibromyalgia can be mild, moderate, or severe and interventions need to be chosen according to severity of pain, level of conditioning, degree of central sensitization, and so on.

Heat and Cold

Heat applied with a moist or electrical heating pad relaxes muscles, increases blood flow, and facilitates healing. Cold inhibits blood flow (while applied) and blocks pain (numbs), leading to relaxation of the painful area by inhibiting the withdrawal reflex.

Heat is frequently applied for 20 to 30 minutes. Cold, using a frozen gel pack wrapped in a towel, is applied for 10 to 15 minutes. Ice rubbed directly onto the skin is applied for about 5 minutes.

Too much heat for too long can lead to swelling or burning and more pain. Too much cold can lead to frostbite. The heat packs sold in drug stores for one-time use (activated by exposure to air or by twisting them) can be used longer, because they aren't as warm as heating pads. Hot whirlpools can expose your whole body to heat. This helps when your whole body is sore. A temperature of about 104 degrees Fahrenheit for 10 to 15 minutes seems best for maximizing the benefits. If you want to soak for longer periods at home, the temperature should be no higher than 90 degrees or so.

Therapeutic Ultrasound

Ultrasound therapy is the application of high frequency sound waves to the body. Ultrasound treatment sets up a high frequency vibration in the muscle/tendon or ligament, generating a deep heat. This brings blood to the area, relaxing the muscles and facilitating healing. Most patients find ultrasound to be a comforting experience.[2]

Stretching Exercises

There are thousands of stretches; the therapist selects stretches that target problem areas found in the physical exam. Stretching is usually a combination of manual stretching by the therapist and self-stretching by the patient. There are many different techniques, such as prolonged passive stretching, contract/relax stretching, and so on.

Stretching slowly is critical. Stretching improperly is a frequent cause of injury even in healthy individuals.

Strengthening Exercises

There are hundreds of strengthening philosophies and techniques. Concentric contraction is less stressful to muscle fibers than eccentric contraction. In concentric contraction the muscles shorten; in eccentric contraction they lengthen, as for example, when you lower a weight. A program that emphasizes concentric contractions with light weights is tolerated best by fibromyalgia patients. Gentle non-painful movement strengthens the muscle by re-educating it to work more efficiently. The number of repetitions is kept low, in the 10 to 20 range so as not to overstress one muscle. It is best to strengthen several muscle groups at a time, dividing the stress on the body more evenly. The physical therapist targets the muscles found to be weak on physical examination to determine what strengthening exercises are most appropriate. With moderate to severe pain, strengthening before complete muscle relaxation is obtained will trigger more pain. In those cases, the physical therapist may focus on relaxing the painful muscles while strengthening those that can tolerate strengthening exercise.

Aerobic Exercise

Getting enough aerobic exercise is difficult even for those who do not have pain. It requires motivation, willpower, and the energy to do regular exercise. Due to the nature of the syndrome, fibromyalgia patients frequently have pain and fatigue with exercise, so they have another hurdle to overcome in doing aerobics.

To understand aerobic exercise, you need to know that the body has two systems to supply itself with energy during exercise. One system initially supplies the energy. If exercise continues, the other system takes over the task. When you start to exercise (e.g., ride a bicycle) the body burns sugar in the blood and/or muscles for energy, because sugar is the most accessible fuel. Burning sugar requires no oxygen, so exercise fueled by this process is called anaerobic exercise. As we prolong the activity, the body switches energy systems so as not to deplete the supply of sugar in the blood, and it begins burning fat. Burning fat requires oxygen, so this exercise is called aerobic exercise.

Nearly everyone wants to burn fat—hence the popularity of aerobics. Aerobic exercise carries many benefits: cardiovascular improvement, increased feelings of well-being, a general strengthening, and the release of pain-relieving substances such as endorphins in the brain. Achieving these benefits is crucial to making fibromyalgia patients feel better. But it's a significant challenge.

Clinically we find that fibromyalgia patients have low endurance and little strength. We also find that activity causes pain. Their muscles are easily injured, so post-exercise pain is common. Their muscles are less efficient than normal muscle. Like everyone, they try to avoid pain and therefore frequently avoid exercise. The key to doing aerobic exercise is in not doing too much—just enough to realize a benefit. For the FM patient, the initial goal involves finding out how to move without increasing pain.

You can figure a basic guideline to gauge *how* much is *too* much aerobic exercise.

First, estimate your maximum heart rate (MHR) by subtracting your age from 220. For example, a forty-year-old person's maximum heart rate would be (220 – 40) = 180 beats per minute.

When you exercise, keep track of your heart rate. Determine what percentage of your MHR you are exercising at. For example, if you ride a stationary bike at a heart rate of 108 beats per minute, that is 60% of 180, the MHR in this example.

Your training index (TI) is an estimate of how much work your body is doing in your exercise program. You figure this value by multiplying three things:

- the percentage of your MHR you exercise at
- the number of minutes you exercise
- the number of times you exercise per week

To realize cardiovascular benefits from aerobic exercise, your TI should be above 40. To keep from aggravating fibromyalgic pain, keep it below 90.

For example, if you ride a bike for 30 minutes (not counting warm up or cool down) at 60 percent of your maximum heart rate four times a week, your TI would be

$$30 \times .60 \times 4 = 72$$

That's within the acceptable range of 40 to 90.

So, let's summarize with the formula for calculating your training index:

[# of minutes of exercise] × [% of MHR] × [# of sessions per week] = TI

It is important to have variety in your aerobic exercise program. Riding a bicycle for 30 minutes uses the same leg muscles repeatedly. This can aggravate leg pain. It's better to use several different activities and therefore spread the stress over many different muscles so one group isn't overworked. A typical routine to begin with is 5 minutes on a stationary bike with no resistance; 5 minutes on a treadmill at a slow, comfortable speed (1.5 to 2.0 miles per hour); and 2 minutes on an arm bike with the lowest resistance setting. Severe FM patients may need to start with more brief periods and a much slower pace.

Generally, the goal is to get up to about 30 minutes of aerobic activity. That can take several weeks, months, or years (in severe cases).[3]

Joint Mobilization

Joints can have normal movement, not enough movement, or too much movement. If a joint doesn't permit enough movement, it is said to be *hypo*mobile. If it is loose and permits too much movement, it is said to be *hyper*mobile.

A stiff and hypomobile joint needs mobilization. Manually gliding or distracting the joint is the usual treatment. A joint that moves normally usually requires no mobilization unless it is painful. Then low-amplitude oscillations (by manually vibrating the joint) can decrease the discomfort. Hypermobile joints are treated with stabilization exercises and sometimes braces. Manipulating a hypermobile joint just makes it looser and more painful. So, it is very important for therapists to evaluate joint movement before using joint mobilization techniques.

For example, the relief you get from "cracking" your neck (usually by a quick movement) is mostly due to the quick stretch of the joint capsule with the concurrent reflexive muscle relaxation. There are beneficial and not-so-beneficial "cracks." Cracking (manipulating) a stiff joint can loosen it, and that helps. But manipulating a hypermobile joint also produces a crack and reflexive muscle relaxation, which may do more harm than good because it makes the hypermobile joint even looser. If much effort is required to get a crack, you are probably manipulating a hypermobile joint and should avoid doing so.

Fibromyalgia primarily affects the central nervous system and the soft tissue, so joint treatment is secondary. Joint stiffness most commonly occurs in the thoracic (mid-back) section of the spine. This area almost always requires joint mobilization to loosen tight spinal joints so the patient can sit and stand properly.

Soft Tissue Mobilization

Soft tissue is composed of muscle fibers, tendons, fascia, and ligaments. Muscle fibers are like cables wrapped in fascia (connective tissue much like a nylon stocking) into bundles. These bundles of muscle fibers are themselves bundled within fascia to form a muscle. Muscles are attached to bone by tendons, which are elastic and can stretch. Bones are connected to other bones by ligaments. Ligaments are inelastic and not meant to stretch; they should limit the range of joint movement so that the connected bones don't come out of joint. Joint capsules are similar to an elastic bandage that holds bones together but allows them to move.

Any of these structures can develop "trigger points." Dr. Janet Travell defines a trigger point as "a focus of hyperirritability."[4] All these structures have pain-sensing nerve endings in them, so trigger points cause pain. Fibromyalgia patients are especially susceptible to developing trigger points in muscle. Trigger points can be caused by resting contraction, micro-injury, poor posture, poor movement patterns, disuse, and immobilization.

Muscles and fascia can also develop knots or restrictions. These restrictions are caused by the connective tissue fibers sticking together and bunching up. Treatment requires soft tissue mobilization/massage to free up restrictions and restore blood flow. The challenge in treating fibromyalgia is doing this without increasing pain.

The following are some guidelines for applying soft tissue mobilization/massage:

- Whole-body massage is usually not tolerated because FM muscles have a hard time reabsorbing waste products (like lactic acid). Massage tends to stir up these molecules, keeping them undissolved so that they don't get quickly washed away.
- Direct/deep pressure causes ischemia (lack of oxygen) in the muscle and usually creates more pain, because part of the problem with FM muscles is they are already ischemic.
- Soft-tissue work should start superficially. Once the top layers are loosened, deeper soft-tissue mobilization may be tolerated.
- A stroke that goes parallel to the muscle fibers is well tolerated.
- Strokes that go perpendicular to the soft tissue fibers are used after the parallel strokes have begun to loosen muscle tissue.
- Using a cream (to prevent pinching the skin) that has no scent and few ingredients reduces the chances that the patient will be allergic to it or have a bad reaction.

Choosing a Muscle Therapist

Most fibromyalgia dysfunction involves the muscles. So, it is important to involve massage therapists as well as physical therapists in fibromyalgia management.

Finding a massage therapist or physical therapist who can help manage fibromyalgia can be a challenging task. It may require trial and error. Asking fellow fibromyalgia patients (at a support group, for example) may help you tap into a network of health care professionals who are a good fit for you.

The following are some guidelines for selecting a body worker:

- Are they certified or licensed to practice what they claim to practice?
- Do they really know what fibromyalgia is—a muscle and nervous system problem?
- How does their technique for treating fibromyalgia differ from their technique for treating healthy individuals? Deep, vigorous massage usually aggravates moderate to severe fibromyalgia symptoms. Full-body, one-hour sessions are usually too long. Direct pressure into trigger points tends to cause flare-ups. Myofascial release or stretching must be preceded by gentle soft-tissue massage.

Patient Education

Teaching fibromyalgia patients to manage their pain and dysfunction is an important aspect of treatment. They need to learn how to manage symptoms outside of the physical therapy clinic. Many patients, and therapists too, approach therapy expecting a cure that ends the need for treatment. It can be frustrating for therapists to treat FM patients if they try to take all the pain away. This results in frustration for patient and therapist and is why many therapists do not like treating fibro patients.

Early in my career, I thought I could take away everyone's pain. A patient would come to me with a long history of pain complaints and failed treatments and I would think, "They have not had me, the wonder therapist, yet. I'll cure them." We both ended up disappointed. I spent all my time trying to eliminate their pain and no time educating them on how to manage it. Now I have learned.

Patient education should address these questions:

- What is fibromyalgia, and how does it manifest itself?
- What can you expect from physical therapy?
- What is proper posture and body mechanics?
- What can you do at home to reduce pain (with heat, cold, etc.)?
- What exercises are beneficial?
- How do you manage your energy level? How many things can you accomplish in a day without pain?
- Who else can you see to help you when you are done with physical therapy?

The Phases of Physical Therapy

Physical Therapy Treatment Protocol

My physical therapy protocol is a guideline that should lessen the challenges facing patients and therapists as they manage fibromyalgia. This treatment regime works best with the patient attending therapy three times per week with a day between sessions.

Physical therapy is done in three phases.

Phase I: The Experience-Less-Pain Phase

This phase aims at relaxing the muscles. The deeper the relaxation, the further the patient will be able to progress in the subsequent phases. Phase one lasts 1 to 2 weeks. This stage of treatment lets the patient relax and experience less pain.

Many patients' previous experiences with physical therapy or bodywork involved stretching and/or strengthening too soon and massaging too deep, aggravating their pain. Then patients were led to believe it was their fault the treatment didn't work, implying that if they had just worked harder or pushed through the pain, they would be better by now. But if they had worked harder, they would have gotten worse, not better.

Typical Phase I Treatment

- Heat application to the most painful areas—usually the back and neck (20 minutes). Those with severe central sensitization cannot tolerate electrical stimulation.
- Ultrasound to the most painful area (8 to 10 minutes).
- Soft-tissue mobilization (15 to 20 minutes).
- Home-care instructions (10 to 15 minutes).

Phase II: Introduction to Active Movement Phase

Most patients are able to move on to Phase II; however, in some severe cases, they cannot and physical therapy is discontinued. For those who can tolerate it, Phase II involves moving and stretching tight areas found on initial evaluation. We start after 1 or 2 weeks of Phase I. The key word is *start*. Often therapy remains a mostly passive treatment. Staying in the warm and fuzzy Phase I is of limited benefit to someone who can tolerate more movement.

Typical Phase II Treatment

- Spray-and-stretch technique to the most problematic muscles (when tolerated) (5 minutes).
- Heat (20 minutes).
- Ultrasound, which may be combined with electrical stimulation of a particularly tight or painful muscle (8 to 10 minutes).
- Soft-tissue mobilization (5 to 20 minutes).
- Joint mobilization, as needed (0 to 10 minutes).
- Passive or active stretching (5 to 20 minutes, depending on patient tolerance).
- Further home-care instructions, adding home stretching as tolerated (5 to 20 minutes).
- Aerobic conditioning begins (12 to 15 minutes).

Phase III: The Strengthening Phase

We start this phase in about the fourth week. Again, the key is to *progress* through the phases. Stopping or interrupting treatment prematurely leaves the patient weak and susceptible to injury. Getting stronger will make the patient less fragile. At the same time, it is natural for patients to want to stay in Phase II, because they usually are feeling less pain and are reluctant to risk increasing their pain.

Occasionally, for those patients with a long history (of several years) or recent severe pain, we delay moving into Phase III by several weeks or months. Severe patients are temporarily discharged from physical therapy at this time and continue their stretching and aerobic exercise at home or at the local gym. At many facilities, patients can use gym equipment in a long-term self-directed regimen. During that time, your status may be monitored to assess your progress.

Typical Phase III Treatment

- Heat (20 minutes).
- Aerobic conditioning, preceded by a few minutes of the patient stretching the calves and hamstrings (20 to 30 minutes).
- Patient self-stretching (20 minutes) of problem areas. Here the therapist may do some manual therapy if the patient is having a problem that day (e.g., pain in mid-back with joint mobilization indicated for up to 20 minutes).
- Progressive strengthening exercises focused on the strength deficits found in the initial exam and/or re-examination. Usually the postural muscles are weak (i.e., the shoulder girdle, back, hips, and abdominals) (10 to 30 minutes).
- Relaxation/posture exercise, such as lying on the back over a bolster for 4 to 5 minutes to reverse slouched position.
- Patient education and home program instruction (5 to 30 minutes).

For a moderate to severe fibromyalgia patient, the time frame for my protocol is 6 to 8 weeks at a visit frequency of three per week. A patient with mild fibromyalgia can progress through the protocol in 2 to 3 weeks. Following discharge, moderate to severe fibromyalgia patients need periodic treatment for flare-ups. These can involve just a session or two, depending on the severity and on how well they comply with their home program and self-care.

We must remember that it's easy for patients to not follow through with their self-management—that's human nature when you feel better. But then their condition regresses. They can get into the habit of relying on physical therapy treatments to bail them out. Also, physical therapy can become an enjoyable experience, so patients may become dependent on it. The therapist must be careful not to enable this.

Motivating people to follow through with healthy habits is a major challenge in medicine. Pain can flare up despite the patient being well motivated and fully compliant. Having a team of health-care practitioners knowledgeable in fibromyalgia spreads the workload while giving the patient the best chance to manage the syndrome.

References

1. Bennett RM. *The Clinical Neurobiology of Fibromyalgia and Myofascial Pain: Therapeutic Implications.* Binghamton, NY: The Haworth Medical Press; 2002.
2. Michlovitz SL, Thomas PN Jr. *Modalities for Therapeutic Intervention.* Philadelphia, PA: F.A. Davis Company; 2005.
3. Clark SR. Prescribing exercise for Fibromyalgia patients. *Arthritis Care and Res.* December 1994;221-225.
4. Travell JG, Simons DG. *Myofascial Pain and Dysfunction: The Trigger Point Manual, The Upper Extremities.* Vol. 1. Baltimore, MD: Williams & Wilkins; 1983.

C H A P T E R
16

Posture/Body
Mechanic Training

Loren DeVinney, PT, OMPT

Patient education by all members of the health care team is essential to managing fibromyalgia syndrome. Physical therapists usually have a great opportunity for patient education because they see the patients several times a week for several weeks.

If you are a fibromyalgia patient, you need to know how to care for yourself when no longer in physical therapy. How do you avoid aggravating your pain, and what can you do during a flare-up of discomfort?

Self-management of pain and flare-ups is discussed in other chapters of this book, so this chapter reviews some general guidelines on posture, body mechanics, and ergonomics for fibromyalgia patients. This information can keep you from aggravating fibromyalgia pain, helping you lead a more normal, pain-free life.

Proper Posture

Good posture is the position of the body that puts the least stress on the muscles, joints, and ligaments when sitting, standing, or lying down. The spinal column is the foundation the body supports itself on. When you look at it from the side, as in Figure 16.1, you can see that there are three main curves in it.

The neck (cervical) region and lower back (lumbar) region of the spine have inward curves. The mid-back (thoracic) region has an outward curve. These curves have a normal angle, which is the neutral position of the spine. Maintaining this neutral position puts the least stress on the back and neck.

If you slouch while sitting or standing, you lose the normal inward curve in your lower back. You also increase the curving in the mid-back and neck area. Doing so puts undue stress on the whole spine, because it overstretches some muscles while tightening others. Also, your head isn't resting on top of your body then. This forward head position fatigues the neck muscles, leading to increased tension and pain. (See Figure 16.2.)

In good sitting or standing posture the head and upper body are balanced on top of the lower back and pelvis, maintaining the normal curves of the spine. This minimizes the stress on the muscles, ligaments, and spinal discs.

Maintaining good posture requires you to be aware of what good posture is and how it feels. Also, you need the strength and (more importantly) the flexibility to achieve the proper position. In many meditation practices the lotus position is considered the most balanced and best posture for sitting comfortably with the least effort—by those who can attain it. Unfortunately, not many people have the flexibility to assume this position.

Stretching is usually the key to achieving and maintaining optimal posture. People lose the ability to attain good posture through long-term slouched sitting or standing. Their muscles become tight, and they lose awareness of what proper posture feels like.

Poor posture is frequently an aggravating factor in neck or back pain. Therefore, posture instruction is a cornerstone of managing fibromyalgia. (See Figure 16.3.)

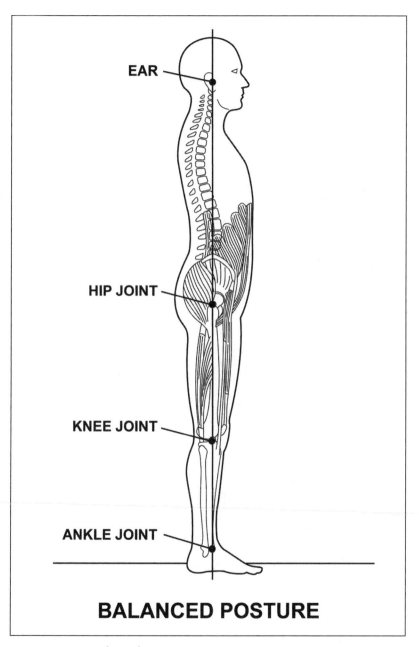

BALANCED POSTURE

FIGURE 16.1   Balanced posture

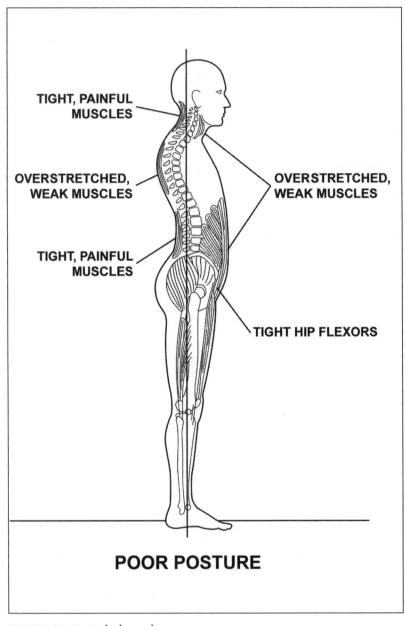

FIGURE 16.2   Unbalanced posture

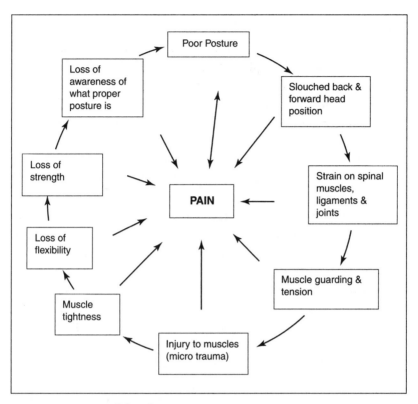

FIGURE 16.3 Painful cycle poor posture creates

Good posture is hard to achieve for many reasons.

- Gravity pulls us over, making the neck and back muscles fight to hold us upright.
- We lose flexibility (for many reasons) as we age, making it hard to straighten up against tight muscles.
- We lose strength in the postural muscles (due to poor posture).
- We lose awareness of what good posture feels like. Often we are unaware of having attained, or lost, proper posture.
- Poor posture doesn't hurt immediately, so we aren't always aware that we are slouching.

Evaluation of Posture

Evaluation of the patient's posture is part of every physical therapy initial examination. The physical therapist observes how the patient walks, sits, and stands. The therapist is also concerned with the patient's posture while lying down (sleeping). If you have less pain in the morning and pain doesn't disturb your sleep, the therapist knows your sleep posture is fine.

Most fibromyalgia patients do have sleep pain though, so a physical therapist must determine whether it is due to sleeping posture or a flawed bed. If patients continue to be uncomfortable after trying to sleep with proper posture, the bed may be at fault. Another possibility is that the patient may be suffering from very severe pain and may need to have some bedtime medication adjustments.

The most comfortable bed is firm yet has a pillow top or memory-foam mattress cover to fill in and support the body's natural curves. Sleeping on your side with the neck and head supported, hugging a pillow to support the arms, and keeping a pillow between the knees is a very good posture. Sleeping on your stomach tends to aggravate neck pain, because the neck is turned to an extreme so you can breathe.

The most common problem in sitting posture is slouching. The easiest way to correct this is to add support to the lower back such as with a lumbar roll. Notice how your entire spine tends to lengthen and become more upright if you support (push in) your lower back (inward curve) and roll your pelvis forward. If you keep slouching in your lower back, it is almost impossible to sit up straight.

Physical therapists look at standing posture from all angles, so we see any asymmetries, like a longer leg or a spinal column curved to the side (scoliosis). We must evaluate and treat these issues individually, because there are many reasons for this problem. We frequently find slouching in the upper back with forward shoulders in standing posture. We all need reminders to lift the sternum (breastbone) and the back of the head toward the ceiling while bringing the shoulders back and down. This corrects poor standing posture. It also helps project a more positive image, something hard for fibromyalgia patients because of their pain.

Often people with poor posture and pain don't breathe properly. They breathe with their upper chest and neck muscles, increasing the stress on these already tense muscles. Using the diaphragm (stomach area) instead allows you to inhale and exhale deeply, leading to relaxation of the neck and body. Notice how much deeper you can inhale if you expand your stomach (push your navel outward). Use your stomach to push the air out and relax even more.

Poor Posture Correction

We physical therapists correct poor posture by teaching posture exercises. These exercises accomplish the following:

- They stretch tight muscles.
- They strengthen weak muscles.
- They teach the patient what good, balanced posture is and what it feels like.
- They provide practice at good posture.

Posture Exercises

As discussed in the previous chapter, your physical therapist does an initial evaluation and gives you specific stretches or strengthening exercises based on the deficits found. The following posture exercises are more general, beneficial to most fibromyalgia patients with neck and/or back pain. Of course if a stretch or strengthening exercise increases your pain you should avoid that particular exercise. (See Figures 16.4 & 16.5.)

Body Mechanics

Body mechanics are the workings of the body in motion. What happens when the body moves out of a static posture? What is proper body mechanics? How can we bend, reach, and lift without hurting ourselves? These are the questions this section aims to answer.

Every time we move, we risk hurting ourselves. A common pattern of injury involves prolonged sitting in poor posture followed by standing up and then bending over to pick something up off the floor. Sitting slouched has overstretched muscles in the lower back,

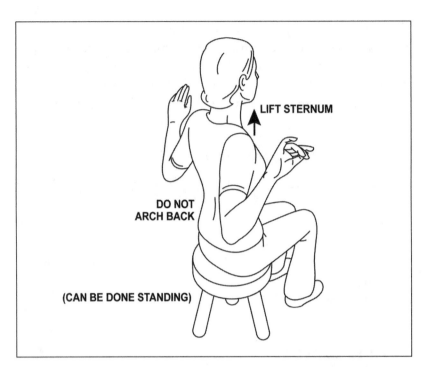

FIGURE 16.4   Shoulder blade stretch. Bring arms up and back as shown. Pinch shoulder blades together bringing elbows back and down. Bring little fingers backward. Keep neck long by lifting back of your head toward ceiling. Breathe normally. Hold 5 seconds. Do 5 repetitions, 5 times per day.

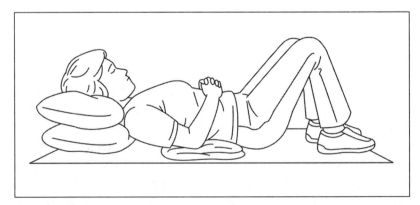

FIGURE 16.5   Thoracic stretch over bolster or roll. Lie on a rolled up towel placed at shoulder blade level perpendicular to your spine. Support head with pillows. Breathe normally and relax for 5 to 15 minutes.

leaving them prone to injury when you now bend over and stretch them even more.

Poor posture and body mechanics has a cumulative effect on the muscles, tendons, and ligaments. Little stresses and strains can weaken them, leading to a more serious injury later. As a physical therapist, I hear daily from patients that they were just bending over to pick up a pencil when their back "went out."

The following are some important principles for proper body mechanics:

- Maintain normal spinal curves (neutral position).
- Bend at the hips.
- Breathe normally while moving.
- Use the largest muscles to do the work (lift with the legs).
- Pace yourself.
- Move slowly and deliberately (focus on the task at hand).

The most important lesson in body mechanics is to bend at the hips. Our natural tendency when reaching or bending forward is to bend at the lower back. This flexes the lower back forward, stretching the muscles and putting stress on the discs (flexible spacers between the vertebral bones) and ligaments of the spine. If you make a habit of bending this way, eventually these structures will be injured.

Yet we are all guilty of bending this way, making it the main reason back problems are so common. To lessen the strain, keep the lower back in its normal inward curve position while bending at the hips. This is how world-class weight lifters pick up massive barbells. The same principle works for us when picking up a pencil or the kids' toys off the floor.

Ergonomics

Ergonomics is the study of how to adapt the work environment to the worker for maximal ease and efficiency. Occupational and physical therapists are trained to evaluate a patient's work or home environment to make it ergonomically friendly. The principles of good posture and proper body mechanics are the foundation of this process.

Computer use is widespread in the home and on the job, so making the computer workspace ergonomically sound is a frequent and important goal with fibromyalgia patients. The ergonomically correct computer setup looks like that shown in Figure 16.6.

The following is a checklist for proper computer ergonomics; each item is discussed in more detail after the list:

- Maintain normal spinal curves. (The position of the lower back determines the position of the rest of the spine.)
- Keep your head on top of your body.
- Keep your neck relaxed.
- Maintain your arms in an optimal position (hands, wrists, and shoulders).
- Alter your position slightly every few minutes.
- Perform posture exercises frequently (every 20 to 30 minutes while using the computer).

The position of the body during computer use depends on the chair and the placement of the keyboard, mouse, and monitor. To main-

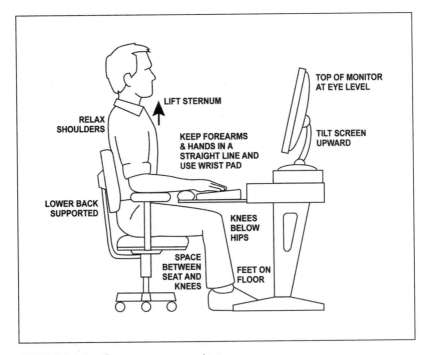

FIGURE 16.6   Computer ergonomics

tain normal spinal curves, keep the lower back in its neutral position (slight inward curve). This is best accomplished using a chair with a lumbar support built in or added. Most office chairs lean back too easily, making the lumbar support difficult to use. Having your thighs lower than your hips allows your pelvis to tilt forward, encouraging the low back to curve inward. A chair with wheels that rotates makes it easier to position yourself in front of the computer. A chair with a high back allows you to lean back every once in awhile and rest your neck and back.

Now that you have the proper chair, it is time to check the position of your head. Remember, your head weighs as much as a bowling ball, so keep it on top of your body, easing the strain on your neck muscles. Imagine yourself from the side. Is your head on top of your body? If not, make sure you are sitting up straight by bringing your sternum (breastbone) and the top of your head up toward the ceiling. This helps put your head and spine in its optimal posture.

Your eyes determine the tilt of your head. Tilting your head back (chin out) leads to tightness in the muscles at the back of your head. These muscles are called the suboccipital muscles, and tightness in them causes headaches and neck pain. Keep them stretched by doing the chin tuck exercise. The chin tuck exercise is performed by sitting tall and bringing your chin inward (making a double chin). Hold this stretch for 5 seconds and complete 5 repetitions. The main causes of poor head position are having the monitor too high and tilting the head back to look through reading glasses or bifocals.

Good arm and shoulder position lessens the stress on the neck muscles. Holding your arms up and letting your shoulders rise up during computer use is one of the quickest ways to give yourself a headache. Using an "ergonomic" keyboard and a mouse pad with a place to rest your wrists and forearms is the easiest solution. Remind yourself to keep your shoulders down and away from your ears. Tilt your head to each side by bringing one ear up toward the ceiling once in a while to keep the neck muscles relaxed, allowing the shoulders to stay down and back. Taking frequent breaks to stretch and walk around keeps the tension in your postural muscles (the back of your head and back) from accumulating.

Conclusion

In closing, I want to comment on several other helpful disciplines that blend nicely with the principles I have just discussed. I frequently recommend yoga, tai chi chuan, Feldenkrais, and Alexander technique. Many other techniques and philosophies will help you to attain good posture and safe, smooth movement patterns (body mechanics), but I have personal experience with these four. Tai chi chuan, Feldenkrais, and Alexander technique have formal, well-established training processes, so you are assured that what is taught has some consistency and quality control to it. Yoga has many different styles and forms. I have found the training differs greatly, and therefore the quality of the instructors can vary significantly. I know many patients (with or without fibromyalgia) who have tried yoga with painful results, so finding a good teacher is vital. I have observed Iyengar yoga instructors to be well trained and to have the knowledge to modify yoga poses (asanas) and movements to decrease risk of injury.

Receiving physical therapy or participating in one of the above disciplines can be a life-changing experience. It can improve your flexibility, strength, and body awareness, leading to greater ease of motion and less painful movement.

17

Self-Management Techniques

Sharon Ostalecki, PhD

How you manage fibromyalgia varies, depending largely on how severe your symptoms are. They can range from very mild and occasional to severe and persistent, so there's considerable variance in the appropriate level of management.

This isn't something only physicians need to keep in mind. Fibromyalgia is a condition where *self-management* plays a key role. No medical expert can know more about your body than you can—if you pay attention to it. Physicians can diagnose, prescribe medications, and order physical therapy, but we must keep alert to any changes in our symptoms, so that the management of the disease stays current with our condition.

Here's one thing that's enormously useful to remember: In recent years we've learned that no disease should be over-treated. *Do everything that can possibly be done* is a poor recipe for fibromyalgia management. Rather, *do everything known to help at your current disease level.* Or perhaps, *do everything potentially helpful in handling your current symptoms.* But, in our desire to participate in managing our care—in our fervor to not overlook anything that may ameliorate our symptoms—we may be tempted to push a physician to take unnecessary measures. (By now, we're all aware of how some folks press their internist to prescribe an antibiotic for a virus—against which antibiotics are useless. Since microbes adapt to antibiotics, using them unnecessarily limits their effectiveness later when they *are* necessary.)

Intense treatment is best saved for when it's needed—if, indeed, it is ever needed. Sometimes, fibromyalgia can be kept at a mild stage for years, even decades.

Fibromyalgia treatment involves the positive blending of both mainstream medicine and alternative treatments. In my opinion, the patient most likely to "succeed" is open-minded. Implementing self-management strategies can have rich rewards: symptom relief and the resulting ability to function at a higher level so you enjoy improved quality of life.

The following suggestions are what I find work best, though certainly they are not for everyone, because we are all unique. In my view, our challenge—yours, and mine—is to "tune in and listen" to our body, discovering what strategies work best for us.

Because fibromyalgia is a disorder with multiple presentations, its management must take multiple approaches. There is no single "tried and true" recipe for treatment. Management varies according to the severity of symptoms in each patient.

The key to effective management is collaboration between knowledgeable health care providers and a patient's self-management techniques. Among the patient skills that matter most is a positive attitude.

This chapter describes skills and techniques that can be helpful at all levels of fibromyalgia. But, keep in mind that this combination doesn't add up to a perfect recipe of self-management for all. As I have said, everyone needs to find what works best for *them.*

Self-management requires not only self-awareness, but also diligence—active participation on the patient's part.

With a positive attitude, self-awareness, and diligence, the resulting decrease of pain and tenderness, plus the increase of strength and energy, markedly improve our lives. Indeed, self-awareness and diligence can lead us back to a normal lifestyle.

Learning

The saying that "Knowledge is power" applies strongly to fibromyalgia. Educating ourselves about the disorder is the first step to wellness.

It's enormously empowering to know what we're dealing with. With fibromyalgia, we must have faith in the body's ability to heal and be proactive about our treatment. The first step to feeling better is to feel capable of taking control of our healing. Understanding the battlefield is often half the battle. As we who have fibromyalgia develop a better understanding of our condition, it becomes far easier to recognize both our limitations and our capabilities.

Ignorance about this disease fosters anxiety. Knowing that it does not damage the body's organs, is not terminal, and often improves over time reduces anxiety about it. There are many books and Internet sources filled with useful information. Ten years ago, you couldn't find a single book on fibromyalgia in most libraries; today, almost any library has a selection of them. Support groups offer just that, support; so do cassettes and videos on fibromyalgia.

As we empower ourselves with knowledge, our journey becomes much easier to travel.

Journaling

Journaling is key to discovering triggers. This doesn't have to be a time-consuming process; jotting down what occurs to you is all that's necessary. The more informal you are, the more honest you're likely to be about your feelings. Journaling is also a useful tool for recording any changes in your medications or dosages, or keeping track of dietary changes and their effect.

In my own journal, I include any new medications—the dose, the time line, any side effects, and any symptom changes. I jot down any new food I'm trying or cutting out. I record the type of day I've had overall, starting with how long I slept and if I slept well or not. I make note of any special stresses, the weather, and pain levels. (I have a friend with fibromyalgia who gets pleasure out of recording every new clothing purchase she makes, because buying a blouse or sweater is her technique for keeping her spirits up. If you use bird-watching for the same purpose, jot down any new sighting. If reading distracts you from pain, note the author, title, and the grade you give the author.)

Journals are a valuable tool! We can look back and see our reaction over several weeks to a change of medication, how we take to a new food, whether we feel better or worse the day after exercise, and so on.

This information, which takes perhaps 10 minutes a day to record, may help us identify not only the source of a flare-up, but also what steps are likely to prevent flare-ups. Information can help us be proactive. It tells us which activities to modify, and which stresses to avoid.

Journaling also helps us communicate more productively with our physician. No one can recall accurately specific reactions to medications, dates our new symptoms started, and so on. Referring to our daily notes makes any doctor's visit more productive.

For me, the most important benefit of my journaling has been to confirm that fibromyalgia is cyclical. So, when I have a painful day, I know the pain won't be permanent: pain-free days *will* follow. I can't overemphasize how this one aspect of journaling helps me keep a positive outlook on the challenge of living with fibromyalgia.

Saying "No"

Learning to say "No" is a healing tool for more fibromyalgia patients than you may think. Most people diagnosed with fibromyalgia are givers; indeed, we prefer giving to taking. It's little wonder then that we find it hard to say no. The problem is that we give all our energy away, leaving little or none for ourselves.

Saying no doesn't have to be difficult. To accomplish it without a negative after effect, just acknowledge the request, decline, and suggest an alternative. Remember, you don't need to offer excuses for your refusal, nor do you need to apologize when saying no. You are not rejecting the person, just the request. This may not come easily to you the first few times you do it; but I promise that the more often you do it, the easier it will get.

Pay attention to people's responses to a courteous "no." Positive people respond with virtually immediate acceptance. Surround yourself with such people. On the other hand, negative people may do everything imaginable to change your no to a yes or to make you feel guilty. What they are doing is manipulating you. The result is that negative people drain our precious energy. You don't need them in your life.

Delegating

Delegating is among the most effective ways to lessen the burden of fibromyalgia. The problem is that many of us are perfectionists and prefer to complete any task on our own. If we don't do it ourselves, we are convinced that it will not be done perfectly. Wrong! We truly need to let go of this belief and consciously begin to delegate jobs.

When I began to delegate some tasks, I was sure it was a squandered gesture—I'd just have to do them over. Instead, I was happily surprised at the result. The work was fine. The truth is that most people are competent and would do well much of what we think *we* have to do. And many folks are more than willing to pitch in.

Please keep in mind that it's not fair to expect people to guess what you may need or want help with. Ask. You'll be doing yourself and them a favor.

One wholesome effect of delegating is that it frees up time for us. We need that time, because we must nurture ourselves. Fibromyalgia is not a deadly disease, but it certainly is no breeze to live with. It takes a toll physically and emotionally. That's why we need to do something special just for ourselves. Not occasionally— at least once a week. The "something special" doesn't have to cost much or require a suitcase. It can be as simple as getting a manicure or having your hair styled. It can be taking off two hours during a hectic week to go to a movie.

In my own life, I have learned to preserve my personal energy for my purely professional responsibilities. I did this by opening myself to the discovery of the everyday tasks that other people are able and willing to take over for me. It's this help—and the willingness to let go of my sense that I alone can do whatever it is—that has freed me to have time to spend on me. Especially on a difficult day, that means time to rest and relax. On a good day, it means time to . . . enjoy.

It's important to be kind to others, and most of us take that seriously. I am suggesting that it is equally important to take being kind to ourselves seriously.

Prioritizing

One of the most important techniques for managing fibromyalgia is to prioritize activities. Most patients find their energy levels highest in the morning and lowest in the afternoon. So it stands to reason that we should try, whenever possible, to accomplish our most important, energy-consuming tasks in the morning. "First things first" is one of the most useful axioms anyone ever came up with.

It can be almost immediately helpful to put into practice the "ABCs of time management." A is something you have to get done; B is something you should do; and C is something you would like to do, but it can wait. If, most of the time, we focus on the A's and B's, we are more likely to maintain enough energy reserves to keep our pain levels low. When that's accomplished, we can attend to some items in the C category.

Try not to overdo it isn't merely a useful suggestion—it's a basic survival mechanism for anyone with fibromyalgia who has a variety of tasks vying for attention. Our symptoms vary from day to day. This means that, although it is tempting on a "good day" to try to complete all the tasks—professional commitments, housework, exercise—on our entire ABC list, it's a mistake to give in to the temptation. Giving in to it will almost certainly require overexertion, thus quickly turning a "good day" into a "bad day." Feeling good on a particular day should be treated as gratefully and respectfully as found treasure—something you don't waste by being an energy spendthrift.

Overexertion always exacts a price. When tempted, remind yourself that this is one of the bad things about fibromyalgia you can control. Whenever we think it's safe to increase our activities, the only responsible way is to take baby steps in that direction;

because if we don't, chances are we'll end up taking a giant step backwards. By going forward at a strictly measured pace, we can avoid a flare-up of symptoms.

In controlling our fibromyalgia, moderation is a must.

Stress Reduction

The number one cause of flare-ups is stress. We sometimes forget that stress is a natural, normal force that's part of everyone's life; however, it affects people differently, and the range of effects even on the healthiest folks is very broad. For anyone with fibromyalgia, stress is always a serious issue. The only way to manage our condition effectively is to find and keep a balance between work, rest, and play.

Although stress is a normal part of life, for us it is likely to arise from the simplest daily routines. "Merely" living with chronic pain is in itself a constant source of stress.

It's also natural for anyone with a chronic condition to have some negative thoughts. And these thoughts bring additional stress. A recent study reported that most people in chronic pain have hundreds of negative thoughts a day, and 95% of these are repeat thoughts. Because negative thinking increases pain, we need to replace any negative thoughts with pleasant, positive affirmations.

Sometimes, changes in environmental factors (such as noise, temperature, and weather exposure) can cause stress and exacerbate the symptoms of fibromyalgia, and these factors need to be modified. Many patients report that sticking to a schedule is beneficial; that is one reason why vacations are difficult for many of us—which makes it all the more urgent to develop everyday tools for dealing with ongoing stress.

Probably the best tool is taking time out of each day to let go of the demands of that day. Simple, but not easy for anyone with the type A personality so many of us have. For us, relaxing an hour every afternoon is as far-fetched as taking a month-long vacation in Tahiti. Hard as taking the time is, harder still is letting go enough to relax.

But there may be nothing as effective in managing our disease as acquiring relaxation skills. There are numerous ways to do this: Biofeedback, yoga, meditation, and tai chi are all techniques that may help you relax. What you *do* then is up to you: listen to music you enjoy; watch a comedy DVD; read one of that little pile of books you haven't found time for (till now); or just plain "rest."

Some of us may need the assistance of a clinical psychologist who deals with chronic pain to help us develop stress-management techniques. If you're among the folks who could use this help, do get it.

Support Groups

If you aren't already participating in a support community, find one and join it. Many groups have monthly speakers, and members share their success with medications, coping strategies, and professional resources. There are also Internet groups for those unable to attend meetings. The National Fibromyalgia Association (www.fmaware.org) provides a list of support groups throughout the United States.

The help you can reap will vary, of course, depending on how positive the attitudes of the group's participants are. Keep in mind that if one group doesn't work for you, it's worth going a little out of your way to find another. In the long run, participating in a fibromyalgia group that works well can be enormously helpful and therapeutic. Also, you will have an opportunity to share what your own experience has taught you, and helping others is among the best therapies there is.

The Basics Summarized

So there you have it. Let's summarize the basics of managing fibromyalgia:

- There is no known cure for fibromyalgia, but the symptoms can be managed.
- Managing fibromyalgia is a process that involves making wise choices and changes that will positively affect your overall health.
- The optimum treatment of fibromyalgia is, therefore, a classic blend of the efforts of the patient and the doctor.

- Self-management skills are vital to avoiding flare-ups and living without pain.
- Whether the issue is pain, fatigue, or cognitive difficulties, patients must listen to their body and adjust daily activities depending on what each day is like.

Remember, you didn't choose to have fibromyalgia, but the choices you make now can minimize its effects on your life.

18

Healing
Through Yoga

Sarah Bates, MA, OTRL, RYT-500

Yoga means "union"—connection, joining. Yoga is that shining moment when body, heart, consciousness, and spirit are all awake, present, and aligned with each other and with the universe. The traditional practices of yoga—a set of ancient disciplines developed over the past 6,000 years—form a network of paths leading to that goal.

In a way, yoga is the opposite of fibromyalgia. In fibromyalgia, the body is painful, fatigued, and clumsy; the heart is sad or out of touch; the consciousness is clouded with brain fog; and the spirit is trapped in an unsatisfactory life. Every part is pulling in a different direction.

Yoga practice gives us tools to relate to our body and life in a new way, a way healthier for the body, happier for the heart, clearer for the head, and more peaceful for the spirit.

Yoga can be practiced by people with mild, moderate, or severe fibromyalgia. In this chapter, I explain how to begin the practice of yoga at each level.

How and Why Yoga Helps Relieve Fibromyalgia

Leading medical authorities now recognize fibromyalgia pain as involving central sensitization, a malfunction of the pain processing centers in the brain and spinal cord. Unfortunately, this not only causes pain, but also limits the brain from having normal sensations.

The brain uses normal sensations to guide bodily movement and posture. For example, the brain controls balance by reacting to normal sensations from the inner ear, the eyes, and the body's proprioceptors (sensing position) and kinesthetic receptors (sensing movement) in all the joints and muscles. From these combined sensations, the brain puts together an internal image, or map, of the body's position and what it's doing right now. Then it uses that body map to guide our actions.

Pro athletes have exceptionally accurate body maps in their brains; for example, they can sense exactly where to reach up a hand to catch a ball. Normal people have a fairly accurate body sense. But for people with fibromyalgia, the body sense is distorted by pain. We can't quite feel where our bodies are or accurately sense our rate of movement. So we are "clumsy." We drop things and bump into things, frequently injuring ourselves.

Repetitive movements and exercise in poor alignment cause pain, which leads to exercise-related flares (sudden worsening of fibromyalgia symptoms). So we become afraid to move and exercise. Then we ache, because the tissues are deprived of oxygen by low muscle tone and immobility. All this pain makes us afraid to use our bodies. We become tense and anxious, so we move clumsily and re-injure ourselves. We curl up in a protective fetal position to sleep or support ourselves with numerous pillows, never lying flat to fully open the chest. Doing this contributes to shallow breathing, which in turn contributes to hypoxic muscle pain and aching. All this leads to poor circulation, which causes tossing and turning to get blood to all areas. This unconscious shifting deprives us of deep sleep. Fatigue contributes to pain, clumsiness, and brain fog, which contribute to more injuries and even more pain—a vicious cycle.

Yoga can help with all these problems. Breathing practices increase the oxygen supply to the tissues, reducing aching. Increased oxygen to the brain can help clear brain fog. An exercise done slowly with meticulous attention to posture and alignment, yoga postures allow us to exercise without micro-injuries, thus reducing the chances of exercise-related flares. By constantly varying your yoga practice (which is easy to do, because there are many yoga poses, so you needn't repeat the same ones daily), you avoid the hyperpathic pain triggered by repetitive motions. By learning new postures and movements, you provide new sensory input to the brain, thus bypassing the learned pain patterns of allodynia and learning new ways to feel your body. By learning deep relaxation skills, you improve your sleep. Also, by exercising regularly, you improve your muscle tone and circulation, providing adequate blood supply to all your muscles so you can sleep better.

By starting at a simple level, you gain confidence in yourself and in your body. As you gradually but steadily advance in your practice of yoga, you grow stronger in every way.

Practicing Yoga

Although yoga has extensive theory behind it, built over 6,000 years, it is intended to be experienced rather than thought about. The oldest yoga practices begin with the breath.

These breathing practices can be done by anyone, even someone experiencing a severe flare-up or someone with additional health issues besides fibromyalgia.

Breathing

Breathing well is important for the following reasons:

- Mental clarity
- Coordination
- Energy
- Pain reduction
- Mood

Let's look further. Full, deep breathing is important for mental clarity because brain cells and other nerve cells need more oxygen than any other body tissue. Most of us with fibromyalgia describe ourselves as clumsy, klutzy, and frequently injured. Improved tissue oxygenation improves transmission along sensory nerve pathways, improving body awareness and coordination. Every cell in the body burns fuel for energy, and that fire needs oxygen. Hence, better breathing gives you more energy. Opening up the breathing releases habitual tension in the chest, throat, and shoulders. Hypoxic cells (cells low on oxygen) hurt. Breathe well and ache less! Shallow breathing also fails to rid the tissues of carbon dioxide fast enough. As this toxic substance and other wastes accumulate, we feel the effects, which physiologically depress the central nervous system, producing depression. Full, deep breathing lifts your mood.

Before we look at some yogic breathing practices, here are some general instructions on how to practice yogic breathing. Read these instructions thoroughly—more than once—before beginning, or ask someone to read them slowly to you. (See Figure 18.1.)

1. Wear comfortable, loose, or stretchy clothing.
2. Lie on your back on the bed or floor, with your knees bent if that is comfortable. Position your body symmetrically.
3. If you are fatigued or have low back or knee pain, support your legs on pillows.

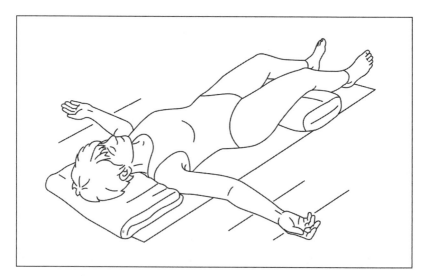

FIGURE 18.1   Supported relaxation pose

4. Support your head with a low pillow that doesn't bend your neck much.
5. Open your arms out to the sides; avoid folding your arms or joining your hands across your chest, because doing so impedes free breathing. If your arms ache, support them on low pillows or folded towels.
6. Lower the lights, or cover your eyes with an unscented eye pillow or a soft cloth.
7. If you prefer to sit, use a chair with good back support so you keep your chest open and spine long. A symmetrical position in a recliner is also acceptable.
8. If you are strong enough, sit upright without using the back of the chair. If very strong, you can sit cross-legged on a cushion on the floor.

First Practice: Observing Your Breath

Observe your breath flowing in and out. Notice how the breath moves naturally, without your doing anything to fix it. Feel the breath entering your nostrils, flowing down your airway, filling your lungs. As you exhale, notice how the *out* breath is warmer and softer than the *in* breath.

You might notice that merely paying attention to your breathing causes it to change on its own. Without even trying to, you might find yourself breathing slower or deeper. It's okay if your breathing changes naturally, and it's okay if it doesn't. Don't force the breath in any way; allow the air to flow freely. Practice observing your breath for several minutes. Then simply let it go and relax awhile before going on to the rest of your day. Or, continue with the second practice.

Second Practice: The Three-Part Yogic Breath

The three-part breath helps you access your full breathing capacity. This is important in fibromyalgia, because lack of exercise, poor posture, and poor breathing increase the pain by depriving the muscles of oxygen. Full breathing is a simple, free, nonmedical action we can take to feel better.

The three-part breath energizes, so practice it early in the day, before your active yoga practice, or any time you need a lift.

Position yourself symmetrically as described above. After observing your breath awhile, exhale completely, letting your lungs empty themselves. Now inhale in three stages: First fill your belly, then fill your lower chest, finally fill your upper chest. Now exhale in three stages: First empty your belly, then empty your lower chest, finally empty your upper chest. Again, inhale belly → lower chest → upper chest. Exhale belly → lower chest → upper chest. And so on.

The first time, do just one or two of these three-part breaths. Then relax and observe your breathing again. Has it changed?

The more you relax, the fuller breath you can take. In the first part of a breath, softening your belly lets the diaphragm draw farther down into the abdomen to draw in more air. In the second part of a breath, let your rib cage expand to the front, the sides, and the back. In the third part of a breath, fill your upper lungs, which extend to above your collarbones.

Be sure to expand your chest by relaxing it, not by forcing it. If you feel dizzy or light-headed, you are probably trying too hard. Relax awhile and try again more gently. If you are prone to costochondritis (inflammation and pain of the rib cartilage), be extremely gentle in this practice. Ease open the spaces between the ribs; don't force the breath in. Yogic breathing stretches and tones the muscles and cartilage of the rib cage, so over time it can reduce the frequency and severity of costochondritis.

Do up to 10 breaths, then relax and let go of the practice. Be still a few minutes with your eyes closed before going on to the next part of your day.

Yoga Postures

Yoga postures are traditional positions that help you develop body awareness, strength, flexibility, balance, and coordination. Often people ask, "Which are the best postures for fibromyalgia?" There is really no answer to that question. A balanced yoga practice is beneficial for anyone, provided that you take into account any injuries or limitations. In this chapter, I cover only practices for people with fibromyalgia per se. Additional common conditions such as neck sprains, arthritis, sacroiliac pain, and so on may require additional precautions. This chapter does not address other diagnoses such as the various forms of arthritis, nor does it address neuromuscular problems such as sciatica or repetitive strain injury, despite the fact that many people with fibromyalgia have these (and other) conditions which do affect both their fibromyalgia symptoms and their ability to participate in some yoga practice. Persons with diagnoses in addition to fibromyalgia should use my chapter for guidelines in practicing yoga, while working directly with a local yoga therapist or physical therapist.

The goals for yoga posture practice in fibromyalgia are to

- Improve body awareness, circulation, alignment, and coordination
- Build strength, balance, and flexibility

Guidelines for Practicing Yoga Postures

Yoga is about inner and outer awareness, inner and outer harmony. Take time on the mat to focus on learning where your body is and what it is doing. Go slowly and hold the pose for a while to feel your way into it. While practicing, breathe in and out through your nose. Do not hold your breath or hyperventilate.

Listen to your body, and don't force it to do anything that feels extreme, "wrong," or painful. Yoga isn't supposed to hurt. Never push a stretch or strength move to your limits, let alone past them. Do less than you think you can. Even practices that appear easy can be challenging in terms of coordination and new muscle learning. Don't expect to master a pose or sequence the first time. Be gentle with yourself and you will make progress over time.

Rest *before* you feel fatigued and you will recover energy more quickly. It's unnecessary to do an entire sequence. Add poses gradually until you can do the whole sequence. At any point, skip ahead to the final relaxation pose. Always end with relaxation, even if you only did one or two poses in a sequence.

Vary your practice to avoid exercise-related flares. Doing the same movement pattern every day, no matter how beneficial, can become a pain trigger as your brain pain centers latch onto the pattern. Vary your yoga session from day-to-day, or alternate yoga with other exercise like warm-water swimming or walking (naturally, with good alignment and good straight-last shoes).

Attending Yoga Classes

The best and the traditional way to learn yoga is with a teacher, one-on-one or in a class.

It is important that beginners with fibromyalgia avoid the faster-moving styles of yoga like *flow* or *ashtanga*, because they go too quickly for our sensory systems to keep up with and we may get hurt. Choose classes taught in a style that has you do one pose and stay in it a few moments, then watch the teacher show or explain the next pose in detail before doing it. Find classes designated as "gentle."

For People Experiencing Severe Flare-ups or New to Yoga

Develop breath awareness first, relaxation skills second, and mobility third.

If you're too ill to do anything else, look at pictures or videos of yoga practice and visualize yourself doing those poses, then close your eyes and actively imagine your body doing it. Don't worry about whether you ever actually will do it. Just *visualize* yourself doing it, in as much detail as possible. Then visualize yourself doing another pose. Build your visualization skills until you can vividly imagine your body doing these poses.

Why? Because movement is directed from motor centers in the brain, dreaming or imagining an action activates the same brain areas as doing that action. Repeatedly picturing yourself doing something can help bring you just a little closer to the ability to actually do it. This practice of visualization begins to create a mental image of your body as healthy and able. It also improves your mental concentration skills, which is one of the traditional goals of yoga.

To begin actually gaining mobility, learn a practice done entirely while lying on the floor or a bed. When you start feeling a little better, learn a chair yoga practice or take a "gentle" yoga class.

For People Experiencing Moderate Flare-ups, Recovering from Severe Flare-ups, Stable with Some Symptoms, or with Some Yoga Experience

Yoga isn't supposed to hurt. If you are grinding your teeth to get through, something is wrong. You may be misaligned, you may be breathing poorly, or you may be trying to force your body before it is ready. Always start the movement from your center of gravity (just below the belly button). Then let the movement roll through your body. Build alignment first (cat cow pose), sensory awareness second (mountain pose), coordination third (mountain pose), strength fourth (downward dog pose), balance fifth (mountain pose), flexibility sixth (standing side stretch pose), and endurance seventh (downward dog pose).

All poses are explained in the DVD *Yoga for Healing. Yoga for Healing* is available from *www.downwarddogproductions.net*

For Endurance

Rebuilding endurance can be the biggest challenge in getting over a flare-up. Part of the issue is that endurance exercises are repetitive and easily become new pain triggers. The secret to increasing endurance is to vary what you do, adding exercise so gradually, in such tiny increments, that your body never notices the increase. This aids in avoiding exercise-related flare-ups. Very, very gradually, increase (1) the time you hold a yoga pose (add one breath) and (2) the number of poses you practice. In addition, if you walk or use an elliptical trainer or treadmill, start with a slow three to five minutes every other day. Each week increase by one minute. If the pain starts to flare, reduce the frequency or intensity of the exercise until the pain subsides. It may seem that you are making no progress, but suddenly, in a few months, you will realize that you have far surpassed your original limits, without ever straining.

For People in Remission—Either Symptom-Free or Close to It

You can do anything you like and go to almost any yoga class, if you observe the following precautions. Rotate your yoga practices and other activities. Few things trigger a flare-up faster than repeating patterns daily.

Build even more endurance by adding swimming or running every other day to your yoga. As with walking, start with three to five minutes and add one minute per week. Avoid, modify, or limit activities that have triggered pain in the past.

That's all there is to it. If you get distracted and lose what you are doing, just start over. No judgment. There is nothing to achieve or prove here. If something other than pain troubles you, anger or fear or despair, just inhale that feeling, and exhale peace. If positive feelings arise, treat them the same way—inhale joy, exhale peace. Whatever your true experience is in the moment, inhale and let it in fully, without resistance. Exhale and let peace flow throughout yourself and out to the world. . . . This is yoga.

I wish you joy in your journey.

Nutrition
and Healing

Sharon Ostalecki, PhD

The doctor of the future will give no medicine, but will interest his patient in diet, the cause of disease.

—Thomas Edison

Good nutrition is uniquely important because it affects everyone—the young as well as the elderly, those who are sick and those in apparently excellent health. Society has increased awareness of how critical it is to meet people's nutritional needs, whatever their age or level of well-being.

The accepted goal today is simple but not easy: to maintain good health, to improve energy, and to optimize mental alertness. All you need do is turn to the Internet or any other media source to read or hear that good nutrition is of the utmost importance—indeed, absolutely necessary—to keep the body functioning normally and make us less susceptible to disease. By now you have also repeatedly been given the message that, should disease develop, good nutrition helps minimize its effects and assists the body in healing.

Good nutrition requires more than a casual commitment. It's not merely a way of improving our life: It is a way *of* life, for none of us outlives the need for good nutrition.

Whether your symptoms are mild, moderate, or severe, eating wisely is critical to maintaining and improving your health. Anyone living with illness should consider a healthy diet as basic medicine. It is certainly an important complement to medication in the treatment of fibromyalgia.

During my years as a professional in this field, I have seen patients experience improved energy and concentration, endure less fibro-fog and fatigue, and enjoy improved sleep. My own fibromyalgia symptoms confirm this observation—eating well has significantly enhanced my own well-being.

Making the best of living with fibromyalgia involves many lifestyle changes. I suggest that good nutrition belongs near the top of the list.

Disease and Nutrition

How fortunate we would be if Edison were as excellent a prophet as he was a thinker. Today, alas, doctors tend to prescribe more, not fewer, medicines than in Edison's day. Still, he was right about diet. And if there are a thousand more medicines to choose among than when Edison wrote his prescription for health, there is also a lot more known about how specific foods can prevent, forestall, limit, or even cure disease.

Right now, there is no medicine with the power to cure fibromyalgia, nor is there any single food that can cure it. But there is no question that what we eat can ease the symptoms of this challenging condition. Both persistent research and personal experience have persuaded me that one reason medical treatment doesn't always help is that, in order to heal, a body needs to call on its own resources, of which sound nutrition is a primary source. There is considerable evidence, both in studies and anecdotally, that a good diet helps the fibromyalgia sufferer to manage pain, which is, perhaps, the most debilitating effect of the condition.

So let's think of nutrition as therapy. Unlike traditional physical therapy, nutritional therapy—using diet and supplements to restore and rejuvenate the body's own healing power—can help a great many fibromyalgia patients deal more successfully with pain, feel significantly better overall, and function at a much higher level.

The plain truth is, what we eat can add to our vitality or sap it; what we drink can help us battle our disease or it can weaken our resistance to fibromyalgia's assaults.

Contributing Factors

Three things make us susceptible to disease: specific genes we inherit, poor nutrition, and lack of sleep. The one we have most control over is nutrition. I am surprised when talking with other fibromyalgia patients by how many place their hopes in a great variety of vitamins and minerals, instead of just using supplements to supplement a *healthy diet*. There's no question that vitamins and minerals foster a strong immune system, but they can't do this important job on their own. The right foods in the right combination are the vital foundation of an immune system in fighting form.

How we eat is one determinant of our health. That's Nutrition 101. But those of us with fibromyalgia need to go further than using basic good sense. I suggest that, for us, changing a so-so diet to a nutritionally dense one is a life-giving strategy. The right foods can not only help us manage our disease, but also help restore us to a level of health some of us can barely remember.

Remember! And eat as though you do.

Wellness

A recent study done at the University of California at Berkeley came to a shocking conclusion: no demographic group in this country—of age, gender, or race—eats well. Americans are overfed and undernourished. Obesity rates are rising hand in hand with disease rates. Most women take in too few nutrients.

For our purposes, let's stick to the diets of people with fibromyalgia. Unfortunately, they tend to follow the rest of the population's eating habits. My fibromyalgia clients typically eat diets high in carbohydrates and extremely low in protein. Muscles cannot repair and rejuvenate without proteins. This is a basic nutritional principle. The overall concept of "wellness" incorporates this principle, among other essential nutritional principles, because it recognizes proteins to be the foundation blocks for building healthy bodies and preventing chronic disease.

What does this mean for us, in our everyday lives as people with fibromyalgia? Plenty. It means that our food choices have the power to affect how we feel and how we act. If we choose to eat a healthy diet, one piece of the fibromyalgia puzzle fits into place.

Perpetuating Factors

Most fibromyalgia patients have what are known as "perpetuating factors." These are biochemical imbalances that make muscles more vulnerable to trigger points and render some therapies less effective or lasting. (These imbalances are one reason why many patients don't respond to physical therapy.) A major example of a perpetuating factor is a diet with nutritional inadequacies. Think of these inadequacies as potholes that pose a continual threat to the machine that is your body.

Hypoglycemia

Another diet problem common to many fibromyalgia sufferers is low blood sugar, a condition known as hypoglycemia. Low blood sugar is the source of many problems in both mind and body. The brain's only source of energy is glucose (sugar). Therefore, how well our brain works—especially the parts that affect our cognitive functioning and emotions—is tied to how appropriately and steadily we feed it. When our blood sugar level takes a roller-coaster ride, the results can be as disorienting as one of those rides. Symptoms include craving sweets, sweating, trembling, shaking, rapid heartbeat, anxiety, depression, and more. Stabilizing the blood sugar level is essential for proper functioning of the entire body. It's only logical that doing this plays a critical role in alleviating fibromyalgia symptoms.

It would be difficult to overestimate the degree to which everything we eat and drink affects the functioning of our entire body. What we choose to consume—or choose not to consume—helps determine the quality of the new cells that are constantly forming as old, worn-out cells die. If our diet consists of good-quality foods and beverages, the body is supplied with the substances it needs to do its jobs well, especially the job of rebuilding cells. If we persistently eat poor-quality foods, we may have increasing difficulty digesting what we do eat, thus depriving our body of the high-quality proteins, carbohydrates, and fats it needs. Years of poor eating habits take a heavy toll: New cells function less and less well, and nutrition-related disease finds a fertile breeding ground in our body. We cannot control everything that affects our condition, but we can control what we eat, and we can eat for wellness.

Let's stop for a moment and see where we are. Say that we're willing to eat a diet that fosters better health, that nurtures wellness. Do we know what constitutes a high-quality diet? Do we even know our actual nutritional intake?

And, most important, is a healthy diet for someone with fibromyalgia the same as a healthy diet for people generally?

Yes, and no.

Diet

The typical diet in the United States is composed of 50% carbohydrates, 15% protein, and 35% fat.[1] Seventy percent of the average American's daily energy comes from sugar and fat—one reason many people live with chronic fatigue and obesity.[2] This type of diet is associated with an increased risk of chronic illness, heart disease, cancer, high blood pressure, and degenerative joint disease.[3,4] This diet is virtually designed for (1) loss of muscle tone; (2) shape, energy, and endurance swings; (3) slow metabolism; and (4) poor concentration. Unfortunately, these symptoms are all common in patients with fibromyalgia.[5]

The basic components of muscle are proteins and minerals. Yet the typical fibromyalgia patient's diet is low in protein, so he or she lacks the material to repair and maintain healthy muscle. That patient squanders the chance to empower the body to cope with, and even lessen, fibromyalgia's debilitating symptoms. In fact, the fibromyalgia sufferer who persists in a diet lacking protein empowers the *disease* instead, empowering it to increase its hold on him or her.

A diet high in carbohydrates and low in protein also causes the following problems commonly observed in both obese people and fibromyalgia patients: lack of building blocks for muscle healing, lack of a transition-fuel source to enable fat breakdown, and lack of a mid-range fuel source (resulting in reactive hypoglycemia).[5]

The 40-30-30 Diet

The ideal diet for a fibromyalgia patient is a 40/30/30 ratio of complex carbohydrates (whole grains)/proteins/fats. When you're calculating this ratio of 40% carbohydrates, 30% proteins, and 30% fats, be aware that we're talking about calories, not grams.

The Essential Nutrients

The essential nutrients for the body are proteins, carbohydrates, fats, vitamins, and minerals. Let's see what each does for us.

Proteins

It is vitally important to supply your body with adequate protein every time you eat. Protein is the only macro-nutrient that builds and maintains muscle. Therefore, it's tremendously important to those with fibromyalgia.

If the body can repair muscle but lacks protein, the process of rebuilding muscle cannot take place. So, a diet low in protein results in more nodules, more pain, and the exhaustion that so often is the partner of pain. But correcting the imbalance between protein and carbs in the diet will result in fewer nodules, less pain, and more energy.

In the 30% of your diet that should be protein, you would do well to make careful choices. Good sources are cottage cheese, eggs and egg whites, fish, lean meats—beef, pork and lamb, low-fat tofu, skinless turkey—breast, ground, deli sliced and chicken—light and dark meat, beans and protein powders. (Refer to Table 19.1.)

For adults the Recommended Dietary Allowance (RDA) for protein is 0.33 grams (g) of protein per pound of body weight per day. This means a 150-pound female should consume about 50 grams (150 lbs. × 0.33 g protein) of protein daily.[6]

Remember: Try to include some protein at every meal. It will help keep your muscles strong. Some simple snack choices are toast with peanut butter, cheese and raw veggies, cheese and crackers, string cheese, a hard-boiled egg, or hummus and veggies.

Another common problem fibromyalgia patients have is weight gain. This is easy to understand if you know that carbohydrates stimulate insulin production and release, and that insulin causes the body to stockpile fat. Since we must eat to maintain energy and health, protein is a much better choice than carbohydrates. Protein helps to stabilize blood sugar. It also stimulates the body to produce and release another hormone, glucagon, which blocks the effects of insulin. Glucagon makes you burn fat, rather than stockpile it, and helps you get off the carbohydrate-insulin roller coaster.

TABLE 19.1 Sources of Protein

Cottage cheese	½ cup (1% low fat)	14 gr
Egg/egg whites	one/one	6/6 gr.
Fish	3 ounces	21
Beef	3 ounces	21
Lean meats	1 ounce	7
Tofu	½ cup	9
Beans	½ cup—cooked	7
Cheese	(1 ounce)	7
Protein shakes	8 ounces (made with water)	~14 gr.
Cheese	(1 ounce)	7
Protein bar	one	~ 14 gr.

Carbohydrates

How do we get on this roller coaster? To find out, we have to look more closely at carbohydrates. The sad truth is that even when you eat them in modest proportion, you can be eating the wrong ones. The "right" ones all fall into the category we call complex carbohydrates. These are found in starches, vegetables, legumes, whole grains, and fruits. Complex carbohydrates provide fuel as blood sugar that the brain and muscles need. It is important—perhaps *urgent* would be a more accurate word—for you to take seriously that even all complex carbohydrates are not created equal. If you suffer from fibromyalgia, you need to choose carbohydrates low on the glycemic index. It is important to understand the term, "glycemic index." The **glycemic index (GI)** is a measure of how rapidly glucose from various forms of carbohydrates are digested and absorbed, from the gastrointestinal tract, into the circulation. Low glycemic foods are favored to limit the rise of blood glucose after meals. In general, the more fiber, protein, or fat in a food, the lower its glycemic index. Typically, both highly processed foods and foods high in refined sugar or flour are highly glycemic.

I'm often ask, "Why do I crave carbohydrates?" I call this craving an attack of the "munchies." It may be a side effect of medications. Many SSRIs and tricyclic antidepressants cause carbohydrate cravings. But these cravings could also be part of a vicious cycle our eating habits generate.

The cycle begins when we eat a carbohydrate (if you're a dieter, it was probably a low-fat version). We feel a "rush of energy" followed by a dramatic crash, which is due to an excessive drop in blood sugar level. Your body screams for more carbohydrates—because you need to raise your blood sugar level to normal. Remember that glucose (sugar), which is transported in the blood, is the only food the brain can consume. That's not only why you crave it, but also why you get grumpy when you are hungry. (It's also why you feel that all's right with your world when you've just eaten something high in sugar.)

So can we break this vicious cycle? Fortunately, there *is* a way, and it's not all that hard to remember—or to do. Always add protein (e.g., nuts, cheese) to your carbohydrate snack; it helps stabilize your blood sugar level. Remember, combine complex carbohydrates, fats and protein; never eat just carbohydrates.

Fats

Finally, we come to the 30% of your diet that should be fat. Like carbohydrates, fat comes in the "good" kind and the "better-to-avoid" kind. Some diet "experts" speak of fat as though all fat might as well be poison, disregarding the fact that some fats are an essential part of our diet. "Good" fat can be found in avocados, cold-water fish, raw nuts, vegetable oils, and seeds. The valuable fats supply energy and fat-soluble compounds needed for properly metabolizing fat-soluble vitamins. Fats also stimulate the release of CCK, a hormone that signals the brain when we are full, which makes most of us stop eating.

Essential Fatty Acids Omega 3 and Omega 6 fatty acids are especially important to the body. In the days of the cave man, food contained these two types of fatty acids in equal proportions. Today's food contains them in a ratio of 10:1 (Omega 6:Omega 3). We need Omega 3's to prevent inflammation, which makes them particularly important for those of us who have fibromyalgia and/or arthritis. A recent study at the University of Michigan showed an inverse relationship between the level of Omega 3's in the diet and depression; that is, people with the highest levels of Omega 3's in their diet had the lowest rate of depression. This was a small study, so these results are not conclusive. But, they may indicate a dietary way to alleviate the depression that so many fibromyalgia patients contend with. There are no Recommended Daily Allowances (RDAs) for essential fatty acids. Omega-6 is amply supplied in the typical Western diet. Sources of Omega-3 essential fatty acids are: nuts, soybean, canola oil, walnut oil, flaxseed oil, and cold water fish.

Unhealthy Fats The "bad" fats, of course, are saturated fats and the hydrogenated oils found in many processed foods. Recent research on trans fats indicates that they may make a substantial contribution to heart disease by raising blood levels of "bad" LDL cholesterol, while lowering levels of "good" HDL cholesterol.

The 40-30-30 diet makes sense for people who don't have fibromyalgia, too. It can improve mental performance and help many other conditions. But for those of us who suffer with fibromyalgia, it is a nearly indispensable aid to a resurgence of wellness.

Vitamins and Minerals

Unlike proteins, carbohydrates, and fats, vitamins neither provide energy nor act as building materials. Their chief function is to sustain and regulate certain biochemical processes, including cellular reproduction, digestion, and metabolic rate. Vitamins and minerals are the catalysts of cellular function.

We need 13 vitamins, 22 minerals, 8 amino acids, and 2 essential fatty acids to sustain life. Without an adequate supply of these vitamins and minerals, our cellular chemistry falters and fails. This leads to diminished vitality, disease, and aging. Since the human body cannot make vitamins and minerals, you must get them from an external source.

Fuel Efficiency

The highest-octane fuels you can put into your body are chicken, fish, turkey, fruits, vegetables, whole grains, and water. The lowest-octane foods are white sugar, white flour, dairy (if you are sensitive to dairy), and soda. Face it, soda is among the worst "foods" in any supermarket. Every can of soda contains about 6 teaspoons of sugar. Our bodies simply don't need any "pure" sugar. Nor do they need processed carbohydrate foods, such as bagels, cookies, white rice, pies, cereals, white flour, and pasta. These foods boost the blood sugar level even more than sugar itself does leaving us with an immediate energy boost, but we feel lousy in the long run.

Unhealthy foods

Chemically enhanced food is properly categorized as "junk food," because we would do well to junk it. Research shows that chemically enhanced food saps our energy resources. Although our body uses a good deal of energy in the digestion, absorption, and elimination of all foods, we use much more energy in striving to metabolize junk foods. That's effort wasted on metabolizing foods that do us no good.

In *Alternative Treatments for Fibromyalgia and Chronic Fatigue Syndrome,* authors Mari Skelly and Andrea Helm quote Joleen Kelleher as saying, "Digesting the normal American diet requires 60 percent of the body's internal energy. If we are only operating at 50 percent of our normal energy today, and we have a normal American meal (which tends to be overcooked and overprocessed and have a lot of sugar and red meat) it is going to take all of our energy just to digest our food."[7]

If we suffer from fibromyalgia, our body is unable to find sufficient energy to complete the digestive process of junk foods efficiently. As a result, toxins have a chance to accumulate in our body— toxins with the power to affect virtually every bodily part's function.

Food Sensitivities

Most people with fibromyalgia also have chronic fatigue. It can be attributed to medications, high levels of pain, poor diet, food sensitivities, and problems digesting foods. Many people with fibromyalgia don't tolerate certain foods, because they cause GI and systemic symptoms. The wrong foods can affect health in many ways. Not only are they difficult to digest, but they also contain ingredients that stress the body and even cause toxic reactions within it. By understanding what's in the foods we choose and how different foods affect us, we can initiate changes in our eating patterns that may affect our energy level, mood, physical stamina, and risk of several diseases.

Ideally, one should feel better after eating, not worse. A small percentage of the healthy adult population suffers from adverse reactions to foods, but the percentage is much higher in the fibromyalgia population.[8] In fact, food sensitivity is a common complaint among us. Food intolerance or sensitivity can lead to, or aggravate, many unpleasant conditions, including constipation, diarrhea, fatigue, joint pain, migraine, nausea, pain or increased pain, and heart palpitations. Together, many of these reactions are diagnosed as irritable bowel syndrome.

The foods most commonly found to cause sensitivities are dairy products, gluten, and sugar (which contributes to reactive hypoglycemia). Most people are familiar with the use of "lactate" to increase tolerance to dairy; some severely affected people need to eliminate dairy products completely from their diet. Gluten is a bit more difficult. Gluten is a protein found in all grains (including millet and spelt) that can cause sensitivity or absorption problems in the small intestine. Sources of gluten include wheat, barley, oats, rye, bread, pasta, and pizza. Most nutritionists agree that gluten is not present in rice, white or sweet potatoes, and corn. Your physician can perform a blood test, called a Gluten Antibody Test, to check for gluten sensitivity.

The Elimination Diet

There is no medical test to rule out food sensitivities, so most dieticians and nutritionists recommend the elimination diet. This is a very simple process: You eliminate the suspected food from your diet for 10–14 days and then slowly reintroduce it to your diet. I suggest keeping a journal of how you feel as you reintroduce each food. If you develop any of the symptoms of food intolerance enumerated above, you may have a food sensitivity and need to eliminate that food from your diet. You can do this with any food, not just dairy or gluten. Some people have sensitivities to vegetables of the nightshade family, which includes white potatoes, eggplant, peppers, and tomatoes. It is definitely worth the time and effort to determine foods you may be sensitive to.

Supplements

The RDAs for vitamins and minerals are designed to prevent overall symptoms of deficiency. They don't give (1) the optimum levels for use by those with chronic illness or (2) the levels required to support healing.

There is no "cookbook recipe" of dietary supplements for those with fibromyalgia and chronic fatigue, but people with chronic illness may require additional nutrients to support the repair process. Medical literature is filled with studies demonstrating that we do make a difference in our vitality, health, and recovery when we eat well and take good supplements.

Five vitamins of special importance to patients with fibromyalgia (myofascial pain syndrome) are vitamins B_1, B_6, B_{12}, folic acid and vitamin C. Important minerals that should be kept in the normal range for proper muscle functioning are: iron, calcium, potassium and magnesium.[9]

In the past, food could supply all the nutrients we needed. However, intensive farming methods, pesticides, additives, and preservatives have made the foods we eat far less nutritious than they appear. Most foods in our food chain contain barely half the vitamins and minerals they contained 50 years ago.

Yet even though the known vitamins and minerals are available as supplements, it's still better to get nutrients in their natural form from food. Supplements are intended to be added to a diet of whole, real foods. Vitamin and mineral supplements supply what's missing in your diet and needed in your body, but they are no substitute for good nutrition. Supplements can enhance the health benefits of food, but they cannot do the job alone. A healthy diet *plus* supplements is your best recipe for a healthy body.

As a rule, supplements should be taken regularly over a period of months. Then the need for them should be reevaluated. People with fibromyalgia often have multiple vitamin deficiencies. In fact, most Americans get less than the optimal amount of many vitamins. A complete vitamin/mineral supplement with 100% levels of vitamins A, B, C, E, folic acid, and D can help ensure that you get a balance of nutrients. Most multivitamins are similar, so there is no need to buy an expensive brand. Take them before meals to ensure maximum absorption. In addition, buy a supplement labeled "USP." These letters on a label mean that the product meets the U.S. Pharmacopeia's standard for dissolution and dosage.

Additional useful nutrients include:

- *B-complex:* (50–100 milligrams) The B vitamins are required for energy production. They assist in the calming process and in maintaining good mental health.
- *Magnesium and malic acid:* Malic acid is essential for energy production. When combined with magnesium, malic acid can be particularly effective. Accordingly, many supplement manufacturers now offer "magnesium malate," which combines the two.

- *Essential fatty acids:* Essential fatty acids help transport oxygen across membranes and act as anti-inflammatory agents. They are found in salmon oil and evening primrose oil.
- *Magnesium:* Magnesium aids in muscle function.
- *Coenzyme Q-10:* Co Q-10 can be made by the body. It is an essential component of the chemical reaction in the body that produces ATP, or "energy"
- *Calcium:* Calcium is a very important nutrient that is discussed in the next section.
- *Glucosamine sulphate:* Glucosamine governs the number of water-holding molecules in cartilage, and is converted to larger molecules that make up connective tissue. This nutrient reduces the effects of arthritic conditions. In addition, for some fibromyalgia patients it decreases pain and sensitivity in the soft tissues (muscles, ligaments, and tendons).

If you take supplements, understand what you are taking and why. Consult your physician or pharmacist for guidance. Again, it is good to get vitamins certified by the USP.

The U.S. Food and Drug Administration has a web site for consumer information on dietary supplements and related topics. Go to www.cfsan.fda.gov/~dms/ds-info.html. The question-and-answer page is very informative. The same site offers a free electronic newsletter from the Food and Drug Administration's Office of Nutritional Products, Labeling, and Dietary Supplements (ONPLDS). This newsletter provides key information and updates on dietary supplements, food labeling, and nutrition issues.

A Special Emphasis on Calcium Supplements

It used to be called a "silent killer," but today there's so much noise about osteoporosis that it's hard to ignore the problem. Still, many women I talk with, at lectures and in my practice, do not take in enough calcium. Calcium is found in virtually every organ, tissue, and cell. Very few major biological activities do not involve calcium's powerful and pervasive presence. Calcium is especially important to people with fibromyalgia, because a low blood-calcium level can cause muscle cramps, muscle tremors, and muscle twitching.

Less than half of all Americans consume enough calcium. Teens are the worst. On average, American women consume 500–600 milligrams of calcium daily. This is about half the amount currently recommended. For adolescents and teens still building bone, the recommended level is 1,300 milligrams daily. For adults to age 50, the recommended level is 800–1,000 milligrams daily. For adults beyond age 50, the recommended level is 1,200 milligrams daily. This level helps minimize bone loss in later years and keeps osteoporosis in check.

If you don't get at least three daily servings of high calcium foods, such as yogurt, cheese, calcium fortified juices, or milk, consider taking a supplement that contains at least 600 milligrams of calcium to reach your daily goal.

There are many types of calcium supplements on the market:

- *Calcium carbonate* is the most economical; however, only 25–30% of it is absorbed by our body. Some people complain of bloating and gas with this type of calcium supplement. To make sure calcium carbonate is absorbed properly, take it with food. Brand names of calcium carbonate are Caltrate, Tums, and the calcium candy Viactiv.
- *Calcium citrate* has a 55% absorption rate and the fewest GI side effects. It is best for those over age 50 or those taking drugs that block stomach acid production (e.g., Prilosec and Prevacid), because it doesn't require acid for absorption. Citracal + D is one brand name.
- *Calcium lactate* has a 45–50% absorption rate and is another good choice for older adults, because it has few GI side effects. But it is very expensive. Calcium lactate is available through Puritan's Pride and Standard Process (they also offer a powdered form).

In addition, vitamin D is essential for proper calcium absorption. Make sure your supplement has 400 IU of vitamin D. Good vitamin D sources in foods are egg yolks and cod liver oil. To help ensure maximum absorption, take your supplements with food and take no more than 500 milligrams at a time.

A Final Note

Fibromyalgia is a condition that has multiple causes. The puzzle of this disease is large, complex, and delicately intertwined. Nutrition is the key to part of the puzzle. We must acknowledge that we all have the amazing power to help ourselves. Once we do, wellness awaits!

References

1. Veigl V. Nutrition. In: Placzek J, Boyce D, eds. *Orthopaedic Physical Therapy Secrets*. 2nd ed. St. Louis, MO: Mosby, Inc; 2006:275.
2. Drewnowski A. Energy intake and sensory properties of food. *Am J Clinical Nutrition*. 1995;62:1081S-1085S.
3. Frazao E. *The American Diet: Health and Economic Consequences*. U.S. Dept. Agr. Econ. Res. Serv., AIB-711, Feb.1995.
4. Frazao E. *The American Diet: A Costly Health Problem*. Food Review. U.S. Dept. Agr., Econ. Res. Serv., Vol. 19, No. 1: 2-6, Jan.-Apr. 1996.
5. Daoust J, Daoust G. *40-30-30 Fat Burning Nutrition*. Upper Saddle River, NJ: Wharton Publishing; 1996:32.
6. Insel P, Turner R, Ross D. *Discovering Nutrition*. Sudbury, MA: Jones and Bartlett Publishing, 2006:222-223.
7. Skelly M, Helm A. *Alternate Treatments for Fibromyalgia & Chronic Fatigue Syndrome*. Alameda, CA: Hunter House Inc., 1999:120.
8. Waterhouse JC. *Food Allergy/Sensitivity: The Pulse Test and Other Strategies*. CISRA's Synergy Health Newsletter, Issue 5, Vol. 2(2), Summer/Fall, 1999.
9. Simons DG, Travell JG. *Myofascial Pain & Dysfunction: The Trigger Point Manual—The Upper Extremities*. 2nd ed. Baltimore, MD: Williams & Wilkins, 1983:114.

20

Journey to Motherhood

Gina Hutter

*Gina and her husband Nicholas lives in Texas. They are
the parents of Isabella and Jacob. Gina is an active member
in her local moms club, swims, and enjoys making
personalized special occasion cards.*

— •◆• —

"Don't try to carry anything too heavy," Nick said with concern in
his voice as I got out of the car, my muscles aching from the four-
and-a-half-hour drive from Detroit.

"I won't," I said stretching, "I promise. Just the light stuff."

He led the way up a flight of stairs to our new home in this
booming suburb of Chicago.

"Well, we're here," I said, scanning the white walls and beige
carpet, tired but excited to begin the adventure ahead of us.

Not that I looked forward to the days of hard work unpacking
and organizing our belongings, let alone the immediate task of

unloading the necessities—bed, couch, phone, some clothes, and cooking utensils. When you have fibromyalgia, a job like that seems like a mountain to climb. But I was up for it.

Afterwards, instead of taking time to recover from the work of moving, I focused on getting to know the Windy City. That must have taken more energy than I anticipated. I know it took more time than I anticipated, including time away from my stretching routine, so my fibromyalgia pain worsened.

I had to find new doctors. After weeks of searching, I found a doctor covered by my insurance who had treated fibromyalgia (FM) patients. He was quick to give me a prescription for physical therapy. I knew how important it is to find a therapist familiar with FM and started calling those in my insurance plan. I tracked down a physical therapy group whose therapists were supposed to have experience working with fibromyalgia patients. With high expectations, I arrived for my first session.

"What can we help you with? Where do you feel pain?" the therapist asked, peering at me over her glasses and ready to take notes.

I had already filled out a questionnaire, giving a lengthy report that I was sure she had at least glanced over.

"Well," I began, "my pain is mostly in my neck, shoulder, and upper back. The left side hurts the most." I hesitated, then said, "I have fibromyalgia, so the pain kind of moves around."

Sure enough, at the sound of the F-word, she glanced up from her note taking and subtly rolled her eyes. "So, you have shoulder and back pain," she sighed.

I wanted to say, "No, I have fibromyalgia," but didn't. Instead, I pushed on saying, "I also occasionally have pain in my hands, a tingling or sometimes numbing sensation that travels up my arms and sometimes in my feet. And I have TMJ. . . ." I continued running down the list of usual complaints, all the while realizing that this therapy group would be a challenge.

Then she moved me to an open area in the middle of the main room to begin stretching exercises. Athletes probably don't mind such a setting, but there was no privacy here. This PT center was in a strip mall. The front and side walls were glass, covered only by plastic blinds. The areas for counseling, massage, stretching, heat therapy, and so forth were sectioned off by partition walls pieced together with a half-inch gap between them that anyone could see through. Not a comfortable setting for therapy one must get partially undressed for.

"This is a neck stretch that I would like you to start with," she said. "It's simple. Keep your shoulders straight, and slightly tilt your head to one side, then the other."

"I know this one, but I'm past it with the stretches I do at home already."

She stopped and gave me a look. "I understand, but I want you to start with something simple. Then, as you progress, I'll have more complicated stretches for you to do."

Wanting her to put stock in what I said, I replied, "I'm at a much more advanced stretching level. This will do nothing for me."

As though she hadn't heard me, she continued, showing me another basic stretch in which you place your back against a wall and press into it with your neck and head. So, I gave up trying to get her to listen and just went along with it.

After three sessions, I quit.

I wanted a continuation of the excellent and knowledgeable care I had received in Michigan, but I didn't have the time or resources to find it. Though that saddened me, there was good news on another front: I thought I might be pregnant.

This wasn't a complete surprise, because my husband and I had recently begun trying to get pregnant. The idea of having a baby grow inside me was exhilarating. What's more, I was weary of adjusting my life to the constraints of fibromyalgia; adjusting to something positive was a welcome change.

I couldn't help taking a trip to the local baby supply store, where I explored the amazing array of products a baby could use. My favorite section was the bedding section. While I stood there picking my favorites for a boy and a girl, an older woman passed by and commented on her favorite, "I like the jungle set. It would be so cute for my grandson."

"Yes," I agreed. "The zebras would really grab his attention too."

"Are you here to pick out a gift?"

"No, my husband and I are expecting."

"Well, congratulations! Children are wonderful. You'll love being a parent."

From there I floated into the toy section, happy to have something exciting and new coming into our lives.

But, as it turned out, the adjustment wasn't entirely positive. I wasn't given a choice *between* pregnancy and fibromyalgia. Being pregnant *with* fibromyalgia was a whole new story, the story I want to share with you.

Help Wanted

Though my probable pregnancy was no surprise, the struggle I soon found myself in was, as I tried to find out what to expect or look out for, given my fibromyalgia.

First, because of a change in my insurance plan, I needed a new internist. With unaccustomed casualness, I randomly chose one with offices at the hospital down the road. I would be getting a gynecologist soon, I figured; for now, I just needed to confirm that I was pregnant.

Waiting in the exam room, I had a list of questions running through my head: *How far along am I? Can I continue my medications? What do I do next?* In addition to such obvious questions, two others dominated my thoughts: *Will my FM affect the baby? And how will this pregnancy affect my fibromyalgia?*

Of course, I had to wait a few days for confirmation of the test results, but the doctor was willing to answer my routine questions right then.

"I'm taking the sleep medication Ambien and an anti-inflammatory, should I continue?"

"Why are you taking that?"

Having already filled out a lengthy questionnaire noting my diagnosis of fibromyalgia and the medications I was taking, I was frustrated at having to explain everything for him and wondered if he had even bothered to look at my chart.

"I have fibromyalgia. I'm concerned how this could affect the baby if I am indeed pregnant and how a pregnancy could affect me too."

"Don't continue to take the Ambien or the anti-inflammatory. Once we've confirmed the pregnancy, you can contact the Ob/Gyn to set up your first appointment."

I hate it when people do that. But, having already dealt with doctors who avoid the issue of fibromyalgia, I shouldn't have been surprised. Then (of all things) he asked if I had any other questions. I replied that I did not (at least not for him).

Disappointed as I was, I was determined to remain positive. If this doctor would be of no help when it came to any possible problems due to my fibromyalgia, I would make sure to find a gynecologist who had experience with FM.

Having learned through the years how hard it is to find an internist with experience in FM, I was nonetheless unprepared for what I now discovered—that it's nearly impossible to find an Ob/Gyn with such experience! After days of relentless Internet searches and phone calls, I found one who had no experience but was open-minded and willing to address my pain—"if the need arises," she said.

So Far, So Good

I'd been dealing with fibromyalgia and its effects on my life for some time, and I was ready to realize that the person who knows my body and its responses best is me. This was a comfort, but I would have liked a treatment "partner" whose clinical experience with fibromyalgia made her empathetic and supportive. Then again, I would soon be taking care of another human being, and looking after both of us during my pregnancy would be good practice. I patted myself on the back—and on the tummy—for my good attitude.

As my first trimester unfolded, I noticed a gradual increase in pain. I suspected that this wasn't a routine development, so I set about informing myself about my situation. I was sure I'd find relevant information on the Internet, but repeated searches turned up nothing. Occasionally, I came across a posting by someone looking for similar information, but no reply was ever posted. I have to admit that this disheartened me, but my first scheduled Ob/Gyn visit was coming, exactly three months into the pregnancy. I prepared to ask questions so clearly that they would have to elicit clear answers.

In about my eighth week, the pregnancy hormones started to kick in, and I began to feel better. By the time of my first visit, I had no morning sickness, though, to my delight, my belly was expanding. I met with the Ob/Gyn, and we discussed all the normal aspects of pregnancy. Since everything was going well, she did not want to pursue any possible difficulties related to fibromyalgia. Since I felt better, I didn't push the subject and agreed that we would take things one step at a time, addressing any FM needs as they arose.

While she was busy checking over her paperwork, I took the chance to look her over. Slightly plump with brown hair and little make-up, she was pretty without trying to be. She had a relaxed and educated manner. Looking up from her papers, she said, "If you find you are having any pain associated with fibromyalgia that you can't seem to deal with, then we can try something to help you out."

She smiled warmly, and I said to myself that she was the first physician I had met since the move who tried to understand FM and was willing to work with me. This looked like the best situation I was going to find. Besides, I was feeling better.

One Day at a Time

As the weeks passed, my pain returned to the tolerable level it was at prior to pregnancy. Forsaking ibuprofen, I took Tylenol when I wasn't feeling well, ate healthy foods, and continued stretching exercises. This no-frills regimen kept the pain under control. Among my blessings is a very understanding husband, who was especially nurturing during my pregnancy. I also had a great boss who likewise suffers from fibromyalgia and showed that he cared by frequently asking how I felt. Though I didn't take him up on it, I really appreciated his offer to lighten my schedule and work load. He was good about an occasional sick day and giving me time off for doctor visits, which made things more bearable all around. I made a point of continually reminding myself how fortunate I was in the people around me daily.

As I've said, I have learned that the best expert on my body is me. To show you how important self-knowledge is, I need to tell you how I became a serious student of my body, its changing condition, and its responses.

From the Top

Back during the otherwise pleasant summer of 1996, I had suddenly felt cramping in my left shoulder and on that side of my neck, as though a knot there was fighting for space. That's my earliest recollection of fibromyalgia.

At first, I attributed the pain to my job, in which I spent eight hours a day at a computer, mostly on the phone as a customer service agent for a major airline. Attached to my work zone by my headset, which was attached to the phone, I was rarely able to change position. I couldn't even stand up to stretch between calls, because as soon as I did, another call would buzz in and I'd have to sit back down to type. I resorted to jamming an empty soda bottle between my back and the chair for some relief. During my breaks, I stretched and massaged my neck. When the cramping was severe enough to distract me from my work, I took aspirin. Initially, the neck and shoulder pain wasn't always bad; in fact, for brief periods it went away.

Gradually, over the next few years, new symptoms arose. The neck pain worsened, spreading up to my left temple and down to that shoulder blade. Then my right side began to mirror the left. I felt tingling in my hands, then a sharp pain in my arms that sometimes throbbed. My fingers began to hurt as if I had developed arthritis in them—a possibility because I spent so much time at the computer. But then my jaw started to hurt, and even my teeth ached. I later learned that this was a distinct but related problem known as temporomandibular disorder (TMD).

Meanwhile, the pain in my neck and shoulders spread down my back and into my legs and feet. From the first, that pain had a sneaky onset, never coming on the same way as the previous bout had or to the same degree. Even now it can be dull and aching, excruciatingly sharp, or like tight knots. Usually it begins as a burning sensation, accompanied by unaccountable fatigue. My left side, the first side to hurt, is markedly worse than my right; but the right side occasionally becomes aggravated as well. Add in brain fog, chronic fatigue, general body aches, chest pains, and restless sleep, and you have my fibromyalgia symptom list.

I sought medical advice from my internist, who sent me to physical therapy. At that time, the pains were gradually getting worse, though still sporadic.

Because of the imbalance between the frequency of the pain and its fierceness when it struck, deciding what physical therapy I needed wasn't easy. The therapist chose therapy appropriate for random symptoms. The result was that the sessions offered only temporary relief.

Both the therapists and my doctor were satisfied with that result. I wasn't. I felt as though the on-again, off-again pain was taunting me. I felt good one day (inevitably the same day as my physical therapy session), and a day or two later the aches and shooting pains returned.

I tried different doctors, who prescribed different medications, including Vioxx, Flexeril, Paxil, and others whose names I've forgotten. Every time I had a severe flare-up, I went to a new physical therapist and sometimes a new doctor. To date I have worked with eight therapists and many doctors.

A pattern emerged: The new doctor would make a suggestion. When it didn't work, he would send me to a specialist. The specialist would study the file, examine me, and conclude that nothing was wrong with me. The implication was that, if something *was* wrong, its center was above my neck.

It is indescribably frustrating to be told repeatedly that nothing is physically wrong with you while pain courses through your body, your neck tightens, and your arms tingle.

Finally, under the guidance of Dr. Sharon Ostalecki, I was diagnosed with fibromyalgia in February 2002. She directed me to excellent doctors and a physical therapist who understood the specific issues that accompany fibromyalgia.

This therapist used various modalities to treat me. Stretching and exercising under her guidance gave me greater relief than I'd ever had during the years I suffered without a diagnosis. She was wonderful! Understanding my condition was only the foundation of her expertise and healing manner. So I went with what worked and cooperated fully with her therapy, both mentally and physically.

We concentrated on one problem area at a time but never neglected the others. This therapist was a relentless adversary of pain, and together we were eventually able to reduce the pain to a controllable level. Meanwhile, I was taking the sleep medication Ambien. For the first time since I could remember, I was sleeping through the night and not awakening tired. I was feeling better and gaining control of the pain.

One Step Backward, Then Another

Now, two years later, during my second trimester of pregnancy, my stomach grew large, and my back began to hurt more. My posture changed, and the pain in my neck and arms flared again. In my scheduled Ob/Gyn visits, I drew the other doctors in the practice. This was frustrating, because I had to re-explain my condition to each new doctor. So, I didn't get the letdown of doubt or disbelief in the doctor's face just once, I got it repeatedly.

At this time my biggest concern was my sleep position, something I had been struggling with anyway. Sleeping on my side causes severe pain in either my arm or neck or both. Sleeping on my stomach causes neck pain. The most comfortable sleeping position for me is on my back. Of course, this isn't recommended during pregnancy once your stomach gets big. I had to force myself to sleep on my side, changing sides throughout the night.

Still, every morning I awoke with severe neck, shoulder, back, and arm pain. I tried adding pillows, which pregnant women often do with positive results. I tried pillow support under my shoulder, under my side, under my arms—nothing worked. I told myself I simply had to get used to it.

Of course, I had to go without pain medication. But the pain was tolerable, at about the same level as before pregnancy. I wondered if pregnancy's hormonal changes had a pain-reducing effect, but I couldn't find any information on the subject. As my pregnancy progressed, I was plagued by the same things that plague many pregnant women: lower back pain, stomach pain, cravings, swollen feet, and severe heartburn. But I was spared morning sickness and some other common discomforts of pregnancy. So, ironically, people often said that I was lucky or that I was having an easy pregnancy. If only they knew!

In the past, I'd found it easier not telling people about my fibromyalgia. Now that decision left me no honest way to explain why I wasn't joining in the cheering. Having fibromyalgia is very painful and difficult; add a pregnancy and you have twice as many concerns. But I didn't discuss this with anyone except my husband. To everyone else's enthusiastic comments, I just nodded and agreed that I was having a fine pregnancy.

About halfway through my second trimester, I started to feel more pain in my shoulder, so I decided it was time to address that and other chronic pains. I already knew that, at my next visit, I was to see yet another doctor I had not met before. Feeling as poorly as I did at that point, I was anxious about what to say to this new doctor, how to describe my condition and wrap up in fewer than my allotted visit minutes everything I had experienced and discovered about fibromyalgia in the last few years. I was unsure how I should ask for help, what was reasonable to expect, and what options I had. To perfect my anticipation, underneath my anxieties I was experiencing Nervousness 101, my customary apprehension whenever I must prepare to explain everything to a new doctor.

To my happy surprise, the visit began well. We discussed the progress of my pregnancy and what any pregnant woman might expect—both now and for the remainder of my term. Put somewhat at ease by the doctor's manner, at this point I told him I'd had fibromyalgia for years and had felt okay up to this point, but was starting to feel more intense pain in my shoulder and other particularly vulnerable areas.

He listened with overtly waning patience as I described my symptoms. Then he dismissed the pain as "pregnancy pain."

I replied that my neck and shoulder pain was the same pain I had been experiencing for years.

He looked at me steadily for a moment in a silence that made me uncomfortable. Then he said that fibromyalgia is a "wastebasket theory."

The most blatant dismissal I had ever received, that stung like a slap in the face. Was he for real? Pain in the neck and shoulder isn't pregnancy pain! Being overly emotional at this hormonal stage, it took all my self-control not to scream at him or break down in tears.

Girding myself, I tried twice to explain that what I was experiencing was not normal pregnancy pain. "You are just experiencing a lot of changes, and these are all very normal," he insisted. I wanted to ask him outright how he could dismiss the pain in my neck, shoulder, and back as pregnancy pain when I'd had it for seven years. But I couldn't voluntarily bang my head against the wall of his certitude.

Instead, I just looked away, determined not to cry, as he went on to explain matter-of-factly what I should expect at my next visit. At that moment I realized how alone I was in the medical maze and that I would simply have to cope with the pain.

Whenever I had asked an Ob/Gyn in that practice about seeing a specialist for my pain, the idea was dismissed. I was told in no uncertain terms that there was no reason for me to see anyone other than an Ob/Gyn during my pregnancy. I didn't know what to do. Should I call the other doctor? Should I find a different physician? I decided to continue with this group of doctors, hoping that the pregnancy would continue without problems and that the first doctor would deliver the baby.

But never again did I ask for help from a doctor in that practice. I became independently proactive. I did a lot of stretching exercises and purchased a yoga-for-pregnancy book to practice those techniques. Taking one day at a time, I dealt with pain issues as they arose. I used heat and ice therapy and took a lot of Tylenol.

During my third trimester, my stomach grew very large, and sleep became increasingly difficult. My stomach was so large it was also hard to move around during the day. I struggled against fatigue. I spent most of my free time during the day sleeping, yet I always felt tired. I took a nap almost immediately after work, woke long enough to eat dinner and get ready for the next day, then fell asleep for the night, tossing and turning. Whenever I *was* able to sleep with few wake-ups, I did feel a little better.

During this period, the fibromyalgia pain worsened. I also had severe heartburn and pain below my ribs on the right side. To feel better, I used heating pads and ice packs, and I tried to stretch. I continually felt I was running out of options to heal myself.

As you might guess, near the end of my pregnancy, I started to worry about the pain of giving birth. By thinking about things like this, I tried to concern myself with the normal worries of a normal pregnancy, but I wasn't always successful. I wondered what effect all the stress on my body would have. I wondered if it would take me longer to recover from giving birth than someone without chronic pain. As I felt my anxiety rise, I reined in my fears about the pain of giving birth, realizing that in what I was already going through I had faced pain daily and had seen that it was, after all, only pain. I just wanted to get it over with and cheered myself by continually reminding myself that my due date was near.

Still, I now started to worry about completely different issues. Because I didn't know if fibromyalgia is hereditary, I worried that my baby might be more likely than other children to develop fibromyalgia. I worried that I might not be able to hold my baby for long or to carry her comfortably.

With but a week till my due date, I took a leave of absence from my job. Free of the stress tied to my work, I started to feel better. However, with that pressure gone, time slowed to a crawl. I am not someone who leaves things until the last minute, so the nursery was already set up. In fact, everything was ready for the new addition to our family. I was physically exhausted and anxious for the baby to arrive.

Birth of a Baby—and a Mother

My due date came and went. Ten days later, I was happy to be induced. Unfortunately, I had to have a Cesarean section, because, as my contractions increased, the baby's heart rate fell, but my dilation didn't progress. I don't remember much, but I do recall the feeling of being pain-free when the anesthetic took effect. And I remember my doctor asking, "How do you feel?"

"Oh, I haven't felt this good in seven years."

She simply smiled, having no idea that this moment was like a flashback to my prepain days and a dream of my heart's desire—to raise my child and have pain-free days. This moment gave me hope for that future and for future pregnancies.

The rest is very foggy in my mind, which is probably a good thing. I remember my husband being at my side, and I remember when my baby girl was born. I remember thinking how beautiful she looked, how amazing it was that she was moving her hands and feet, and how now nothing else mattered.

The following days were filled with both pain and joy, of course. I was given Ambien for the first few nights but didn't continue taking it after that. For, if I took a sleeping aid, I might not be able to wake up fully when my baby needed me at night. Even though the nine-months' journey of pregnancy was over, I had much further to go.

Though my mom came to stay with us and help out, the first few weeks at home were virtually sleepless. But every new parent goes through this rite of passage—a fact I repeated to myself as often as necessary. Healing from the Cesarean delivery was long and extremely painful, but slowly I began to feel better. When I was finally able to sleep through most of the night, it was a blessed relief. I felt okay, and the fibromyalgia pain wasn't too bad. I continued to feel better as I bonded with my daughter and learned to take care of her needs in a responsive rather than bookish way. A settling feeling came over my husband and I, we felt comfortable. We were now a family . . . in a new city . . . in a new home . . . and blessed with a child.

Now that my daughter and I are adjusting to the brand-new immediate world we share, I find it natural to focus on the pleasure Isabella gives me rather than on my physical problems. Still, it's hard to ignore my continuing heartburn. And though it doesn't steal much attention from my child, fibromyalgia pain is seeping back into my life. Looking back, I realize that during pregnancy I felt mostly the same as before and at times I even felt better. Now I'm picking up where I left off before the pregnancy began.

I treasure the lessons I learned. If I have another child, I won't be afraid or feel helpless. I'll know that any difficulties won't be worse than I can handle; that I can and will cope. My advice to anyone with fibromyalgia who wants to become pregnant—or may be already pregnant and worried—is to take control, to ask for whatever help you need, and to keep asking until someone listens. Yet, even as you look for answers from professionals, never forget that you are the primary expert on your body. Stretch, exercise, take a pregnancy yoga class, eat well, and relax. You may find, as I did, that pregnancy can actually make you feel better for the duration. Your reward for doing all those exercises and asking all those questions is your wonderful baby.

When I was pregnant with our second child, Jake, I experienced similar pains/challenges as with our first child. Throughout the pregnancy I maintained a comfort level by utilizing hot and cold therapy (ice packs and heating pads) along with stretching. My physician suggested water physical therapy, and I found it to be quite relaxing.

I had an easier and quicker recovery with this birth, and in the months that followed I adjusted to having two children and the challenges of living with fibromyalgia.

My second pregnancy, as with my first, was a constant learning experience. I have found that having fibromyalgia requires a constant ongoing search for what can help me to feel better and I expect that my journey has just begun.

Currently my family and I reside in the Chicago area. We are busy enjoying our children and the happiness they bring to our lives.

CHAPTER
21

Importance of Foot and Ankle Alignment in Fibromyalgia

Ernst Bastian, CO

The bony structures of the foot resemble the pieces of a jigsaw puzzle, with bony prominences that fit together. If pieces don't fit, or if the bones are out of alignment, their surfaces wear unevenly where the bones connect at the joints. The result can be great discomfort. Often orthotic appliances can help relieve this discomfort.

Unfortunately, there is no established procedure to guide orthotists in treating patients with fibromyalgia and other chronic pain syndromes. Therefore, we must rely on our years of experience with such patients, which includes trial and error. Not every patient is a candidate for custom-molded foot orthoses. If you have foot pain, first get an orthotic evaluation from a physician, possibly see a physical therapist, and finally an orthotist. After your consultation you will know what to expect from foot orthoses.

The achievable goals for a patient with fibromyalgia or chronic pain syndrome are:

- To restore alignment
- To distribute weight throughout entire bottom surface of foot
- To absorb shock

First, the problem must be diagnosed as either a soft-tissue problem, or a bone-alignment problem, or a combination of both.

If a malalignment is flexible, it can be corrected; if not, orthotic management is often unsuccessful. Even if the pain stems from soft tissue (i.e., fat pads, muscles, or tendons) we must assess the alignment of the foot. If the problem is simply that the padding is insufficient, an orthotist needs only to provide additional padding.

Common Foot Problems in Fibromyalgia Patients

I find three problems common among fibromyalgia patients:

- Poor mechanical alignment
- Insufficient shock absorption
- Poor weight distribution over the bottom of the foot

As mentioned earlier, we must first identify the problem through an orthotic evaluation. Is it an alignment issue, a weight distribution issue, or a shock absorption issue? Unfortunately, sometimes it's a combination of two or all of these conditions.

Alignment

Your alignment must be checked both while you are standing and while you are walking at various speeds (deviations are easier to identify at greater velocities). Proper assessment of the patient's gait is essential in making the proper orthotic recommendation. Boiled down to simplest terms, a normal gait follows this pattern: the heel strikes first, you walk on the outside of the foot, roll to the inside across the ball, and then roll off the toes.

Heel Strike → Outside of Foot → Inside of Foot → Off the Toes

If your gait doesn't follow this pattern, you can have multiple alignment and wear issues on the joint surfaces of the bones. These issues affect not only the foot and the ankle, but also the knees, hips, and lower and upper back. Clinical signs are tired or sore joints, which are often caused by an inefficient gait. Abnormal gait is considered an alignment issue, and the goal of foot orthoses is to restore proper alignment.

Pronation and Supination

The most common gait abnormalities are pronation and supination. In pronation you walk too much on the inside of your foot. In supination you walk too much on the outside of your foot. With pronation we see a more knock-kneed angle at the knee, uneven wear at the lateral (outside) ankle, lateral knee, the hip, and excessive sway or pelvic oscillation during walking. With supination we see more bow-leggedness at the knee, increased medial (inside) ankle and knee wear with excessive pelvic oscillation, and probably a backward lean in the lower back. Again, if these are flexible alignment issues, of the foot, they can be corrected through foot orthoses. If they are fixed deformities, foot orthoses are less successful.

About 85% of us pronate, 15% supinate, and very few have a textbook gait. A patient with fibromyalgia or chronic pain syndrome who pronates or supinates has imbalanced opposing muscle and tendon groups.

For example, if a patient pronates: (Figure 21.1)

- The inner part of the foot, ankle, and knee have elongated muscles and tendons.
- The bony prominences on the outside of the ankle and knee are compressed.

The result is uneven wear and often soft-tissue discomfort due to some muscles being overstretched and other muscles maintaining a contracted posture.

A patient who supinates (Figure 21.2) would experience the opposite effect:

- Elongation of the outside muscles and tendons
- Compression of the inside ankle and knee joints

In short, the body works best and muscles and tendons are in balance when the foot and ankle, knee, hip, and lower back are in as straight of an alignment as possible.

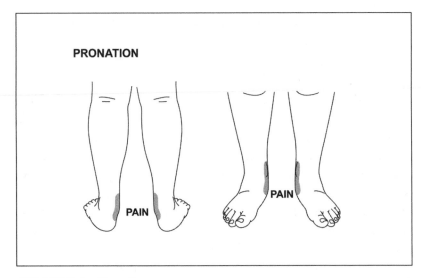

FIGURE 21.1   Pronation

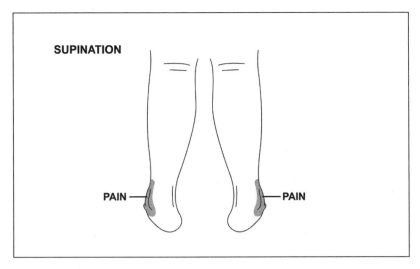

FIGURE 21.2   Supination

Metatarsalgia

Patients with fibromyalgia often suffer from a soft-tissue condition known as metatarsalgia, which is pain in the ball of the foot (at the heads of the metatarsal bones). It can be caused by reduced fat pads in the ball of the foot, poor shoe selection (i.e., high heels) and poor mechanics. In the latter case, the part of the arch just before the ball (the metatarsal arch) has fallen, causing uneven pressure across the ball. As always, if this is a flexible condition orthotics can help. An orthotic can lift the metatarsal arch, relieving pressure by "unweighting" the metatarsal heads. But if the deformity is fixed, the only hope is to pad the ball of the foot, dispersing the pressure and cushioning the foot on impact.

As we age, the fat pads in the heel and ball often reduce. Sensitive people with minimal cushioning are more susceptible to pain and discomfort in those areas, and they don't get sufficient cushioning from their shoes alone. Therefore, the orthosis must substitute for lost fat tissue.

Weight Distribution

Weight distribution is another important issue for patients with chronic pain. Pressure is reduced when it is evenly distributed over a greater surface area. So, the pressure of your weight is most easily borne when it is evenly distributed over the entire bottom surface of your foot instead of in isolated areas alone. Then your feet can bear your weight for a long time before becoming fatigued or painful.

Some people have a very high longitudinal arch, a condition called a cavus foot. The longitudinal arch is the most commonly known arch, on the inner part of the foot. If it's very high, you don't get adequate support from a store-bought shoe. That's because only 15% of us have a cavus foot, and shoe manufacturers market to the 85% of us who pronate or have a flatter longitudinal arch. Consequently, patients with a cavus foot have poor weight distribution in their shoes. Their weight is borne mainly at the heels and balls, with a little on the toes, but with minimal or no support through the midsection of the foot.

Orthotics

Once your orthotist has diagnosed the problem, he or she can make a proper orthotic recommendation. The three basic functions of an orthotic for a patient with painful, hypersensitive, misaligned feet would be to:

- Restore alignment
- Distribute weight evenly across the entire bottom surface of the foot
- Absorb shock upon impact of walking

The dream orthotic for a patient with fibromyalgia or chronic pain gives maximum support, cushions the foot, and absorbs the shock but doesn't touch the hypersensitive patient. Of course, no such orthotic exists. Therefore tolerance becomes a very important issue with these patients.

Often the orthotist must gradually introduce a foot orthosis. You initially wear the orthotics briefly, for as little as 10 minutes several times per day. As you increase wearing time, your orthotist is able to gradually increase the support they provide. Therefore, the relationship between orthotist and patient must be a positively directed one, in which both parties are patient. I say this because it often takes multiple appointments to accommodate the patient and provide maximum support and comfort.

In making orthoses for fibromyalgia patients, I have found that softer is better with an initial orthosis for a patient who hasn't worn orthoses before. Fabricating an orthosis that is too rigid results in poor acceptance by the patient. This leads to frustration for both patient and practitioner. Ultimately, the patient doesn't benefit from the long-term effects of orthotics, and forms the potentially false belief that orthotics do not work. Once the patient can tolerate the orthosis, the orthotist can increase the correction and address the alignment issues. The functional goal is to restore alignment to as close to neutral as possible, allowing an efficient gait and the best possible weight distribution. Then the patient can maintain an upright standing position and increase their activity level to build the muscles also into a proper alignment. Thus, the patient strengthens into a more stable, efficient posture.

The actual type of orthosis we make depends on the patient's

- Mechanical problems
- Stature
- Height and weight
- Activity level/Occupation
- Shoe type
- Tolerance of pressure

Most orthoses are multi-layered, with a soft layer against the patient's foot and more stabilizing material in subsequent layers. Occasionally, diagnostic foot orthoses are used to test the patient's tolerance and to indicate weight distribution areas. These orthoses are highly adjustable. We can easily add or remove padding to discover what makes you most comfortable. Once the orthosis is acceptable and you can wear it for a long time, we make a permanent one that is durable but not as adjustable as the diagnostic one.

Some permanent orthotics are made of silicone, which has qualities that are excellent for the chronic-pain patient. Silicone orthotics rebound, so they maintain their shape for several years without deforming or compressing. Silicone is difficult to work with, however, because nothing adheres to silicone but silicone. So, little adjustment can be made to silicone orthoses. Therefore, you get them only when the orthotist is confident that you will tolerate the alignment and correction.

Off-the-Shelf Orthotics

What about orthotics you can buy off-the-shelf?

As an orthotist, I favor custom orthoses, because they provide a total-contact fit and a more even weight distribution. Patients tend to tolerate custom orthoses better than those bought off-the-shelf. And, through a total-contact fit, an orthotist can provide greater correction and therefore improved alignment.

That said, there are some beneficial off-the-shelf orthoses. If you have mainly shock-absorption issues and minimal mechanical-alignment issues, a well-padded off-the-shelf orthosis provides excellent shock absorption and cushioning.

Off-the-shelf orthoses range from $15–$75 and often serve as a good trial, letting you know that orthotics help. So, you might try a pair before investing in custom orthotics, which cost from $300–$500 per pair. However, poor results with off-the-shelf orthotics don't always mean poor results with custom orthotics. Patients dissatisfied with off-the-shelf orthotics shouldn't give up and assume that they aren't candidates for custom orthotics.

Shoes

Your orthotics won't work if you don't wear good shoes. I tell my patients that orthotics can provide no more than half the support you need, so your shoes should provide the other half. If they are worn-out, flimsy, too large, or too small, then your foot orthoses provide most of your correction and support, and that isn't enough.

Several issues come into play when recommending shoes. We consider the patient's job, lifestyle, activity level, recreational activity, and foot type.

As you've already seen, cushioning is essential for patients with chronic pain. Therefore, don't get rigid-soled shoes with hard rubber or leather soles. Look for a shoe with adequate cushioning that you can compress with both thumbs. If you can compress the sole with your thumb, the shoe will compress adequately when your heel strikes the ground.

The sole of your shoe should be at least as wide as the sole of your foot. Wider soles give you better balance and weight distribution. Hence, high-heeled shoes with narrow soles reduce your balance and focus pressure on small areas of the foot—namely, the center of the heel and the ball of the foot.

When assessing a shoe, hold it at the heel and the toe, and then bend it. It should bend at the ball of the foot, not in the arch. That's because your foot needs support through the heel and the arch, while it needs flexibility at the ball to allow proper function during the gait cycle.

I am often asked how high the heel should be for a patient with chronic pain issues. There is no simple answer. The lower the heel is, the more even the weight distribution. Yet, with a very low heel, many patients feel tipped backward. Therefore a slight heel with a ½ in difference between the height of the heel and ball of the shoe respectively is sufficient and often provides adequate stability. Avoid heels that pitch you forward and focus your weight on the ball of the foot.

Walking versus Running Shoes

The shoes that seem to work best are running shoes or walking shoes. What's the difference? A running shoe has a "rockered" sole, which is sloped at the heel and at the ball of the foot to promote a smooth gait pattern. A walking shoe has a flatter heel and is rolled at the ball of the foot. Each type of shoe is optimized for the appropriate speed. But the rockered sole of the running shoe does offer some help for gait problems, because the rollover at heel strike is important to maintain a running pattern. I personally favor a running shoe, because it has a wider base of support, a rockered sole, and more cushioning.

As an orthotist that treats fibromyalgia and other chronic pain patients, I find this group to be one of the most challenging. 1/64 of an inch adjustment may cause you to either improve or worsen alignment and/or function. The positive patient-practitioner relationship must be established at the first visit, and realistic expectations must be defined. That is orthotic management will not cure chronic pain but by being a "patient-patient," pain may be reduced significantly and functionality increased resulting in improved quality of life.

22

Behaviorally Reconnecting Mind and Body

Donald Moss, PhD

Mind–body approaches begin by recognizing that fibromyalgia is a real medical disorder, accompanied by measurable changes in a variety of biological systems. Fibromyalgia has dramatic effects on the body and the mind of the patient. Until quite recently, many patients could not persuade their physicians to believe in the reality of their symptoms. The term *fibromyalgia* was used in a disparaging way, and many health care professionals believed that the majority of fibromyalgia patients' symptoms were either imaginary or a byproduct of depression.

In fact, fibromyalgia is not new and is not imaginary. It was first described by Dr. William Balfour, a Scottish surgeon at the University of Edinburgh, in 1816. Yet fibromyalgia was not officially recognized as an illness by the American Medical Association until 1987, and as a syndrome by the World Health Organization until 1993. Modern systematic diagnostic criteria were developed by the American College of Rheumatology in 1990, and the current official definition was created by an international conference of physicians and researchers in Copenhagen in 1992. The "Copenhagen Declaration" document recognized that fibromyalgia is the most common cause of widespread musculoskeletal pain.[1]

Mind–body therapies for fibromyalgia include sleep hygiene, exercise, biofeedback, progressive muscle relaxation, neurofeedback, audio-visual entrainment, heart rate variability training, relaxation skills, hypnosis, and imagery training.

The Signs and Symptoms of Fibromyalgia

Fibromyalgia literally means "pain in the fiber of the muscles." The most prominent feature of fibromyalgia is the presence of pain throughout the musculature, often burning, either constant or recurrent, and varying in severity. However, the muscle pain is often confusing to the patient and the health practitioner, because the pain fades and intensifies, and changes location within the body, without a clear trigger. The pain often (not always) begins at the site of an injury, but becomes systemic, spreading around the entire musculature. Over time the entire musculature shows changes, including hyperalgesia—extreme sensitivity to exertion, strain, or trauma, with many routine activities triggering intense and severe pain.

Further, the muscular pain is accompanied by a confusing variety of seemingly unrelated symptoms. Patients frequently report fatigue, low energy, sleep disturbance, morning stiffness, symptoms of irritable bowel syndrome, emotional symptoms such as depression and anxiety, and cognitive deficits such as poor concentration, impaired memory, and a clouding of their consciousness ("fibro-fog").

Mechanisms of Fibromyalgia Addressed by Mind–Body Therapies

The baffling and fluctuating pattern of muscle pain, and the wide range of accompanying symptoms, tells us that fibromyalgia is not a local muscle problem.

Chronobiological Disturbance

One view is that fibromyalgia is a "chronobiological disorder." It involves changes in basic biological rhythms. The sleep–wake cycle is disturbed in fibromyalgia patients, so that patients experience difficulty falling asleep, frequent awakening, early morning awakening, and chronic low energy and loss of interest in activity. Sleep studies show a lack of the deeper delta range sleep necessary to refresh the person physically and emotionally. Many individuals display a serious disorganization of the sleep cycle, with brief intermittent periods of fitful restless sleep throughout the day and night. The resultant sleep deprivation contributes substantially to disturbance in a variety of biological and psychological functions, including brain rhythms and mood.

Muscle Dysfunction

Individuals with fibromyalgia show a number of abnormal patterns in muscle physiology. Stuart Donaldson, a researcher in Calgary, Alberta, has identified several key patterns in the muscles of fibromyalgia patients[2]:

- High basal levels of muscle tension, even at rest
- Asymmetries—higher levels of muscle tension in the same muscle on one side of the body than on the other
- Co-activations—muscles that are not functionally involved in a movement tense anyway during activity
- Failure to recover after exertion—muscles do not relax again following use
- Long-term atrophy of muscle tissue, with shortening of muscle fibers and increased sensitivity

Many of these abnormalities make sense, in terms of the patient's body reacting to the presence of pain. When human beings feel pain, they tense and brace against the pain. Sometimes they will twist their posture defensively around the pain site. Finally, the tensed torso and musculature lose flexibility, and, for example, when the individual in pain moves his or her head, large areas of the torso musculature will tense and activate as well. In addition, individuals in severe pain avoid activity to minimize pain. This results in a muscle disuse syndrome, which includes the atrophy of muscle tissue and muscle deconditioning, and the loss of flexibility and strength.

Abnormal Patterns in the Brain and Nervous System

Sleep disturbance, which is so characteristic of fibromyalgia, is associated with a disturbance in the electrical rhythms of the brain. The presence of excessive amounts of alpha activity (8–12 cycles per second) during sleep is associated with the absence of restorative, restful sleep in fibromyalgia patients.[3] Many fibromyalgia patients fail to reach the deeper delta rhythms (1–3 cycles per second) that mark restorative sleep. During the deepest stages of sleep the muscles are able to completely relax. Sleep disturbance, and especially the absence of deep restorative sleep, contributes to the presence of pain and clinical depression in fibromyalgia.

Autonomic Dysfunction

Many individuals with fibromyalgia show chronic disturbances in the functioning of the autonomic nervous system that regulates many of the internal functions of their bodies. The autonomic nervous system (ANS) is commonly known as the involuntary nervous system, and is responsible for regulating blood pressure, heart rate, skin sweating, core temperature, and digestion. The ANS is made of two parts, the stimulating part, known as the sympathetic nervous system, and the calming part, known as the parasympathetic nervous system. Several research studies have reported an over-activation of the sympathetic nervous system in people with fibromyalgia.[4,5,6] When the sympathetic nervous system is activated in someone who has fibromyalgia, their muscles contract, causing increased pain. Sympathetic activation also provokes the familiar biological "fight or flight response" in the face of threat or danger; this is the body's means of mobilizing to fight danger. However, this sympathetic activation can also become chronic and habitual, producing physiological fatigue, depletion of coping resources, and impaired immune function.

Precipitating Factors or Events Leading to the Onset of Fibromyalgia

Primary fibromyalgia occurs spontaneously in individuals not suffering from any related or triggering condition. There is no clear cause for "primary fibromyalgia," but over time the severity of primary fibromyalgia is affected by factors such as sleep deprivation, muscle atrophy, emotional stress, coping style, the weather, and of course, the pain itself. The course tends to be chronic, with unpredictable periods of greater and lesser severity.

Secondary fibromyalgia occurs in patients whose pain was preceded or triggered by another illness, such as arthritis, bursitis, or lupus, or from abnormal structural conditions such as disc tears and herniations, and nerve entrapments. The course and appearance of secondary fibromyalgia is very similar to primary fibromyalgia. The picture is complicated because the patient's other illness or illnesses continue to cause symptoms and require treatment. It is often a difficult medical challenge to know when a triggering factor, such as a disc herniation, should be addressed surgically or whether other pain control methods should be pursued. A great many patients with fibromyalgia respond poorly to surgery, so it has been suggested by some experts that, for fibromyalgia patients, nonsurgical options should be the first course of action when conditions permit.

Finally, post-traumatic fibromyalgia begins with a specific injury, often one with localized pain. Over time the more widespread pattern of fibromyalgia pain develops and the other symptoms of fibromyalgia emerge. The intervention plan must include treating and rehabilitating the original injury, as well as treating and rehabilitating the individual for fibromyalgia. The patient may also continue to suffer fibromyalgia symptoms even if the original injury heals. This occurs when the body reacts to the pain of the fibromyalgia as it did with the post-traumatic injury, by producing more pain—via muscle dysfunction, sleep disturbance, and so on.

Mind–Body Therapy Approaches for Fibromyalgia

Balancing the Muscles: Muscle Biofeedback

A number of authors in the United States and Europe have published research studies showing that muscle biofeedback can benefit fibromyalgia patients.[7,8,9] Muscle biofeedback uses electronic instruments to measure muscle tension in any muscle group. Biofeedback sensors are placed on the surface over the muscle, and the instrument detects the electrical firing of motor neurons, summing the activity and displaying it back to the patient on an instrument gauge or more commonly on a computer screen.[10] Patients improve their ability to identify and assess the amounts of tension present, and gradually develop the ability to reduce muscle tension in specific muscles. Muscle biofeedback has been shown to reduce pressure point or tender point sensitivity, reduce the amount of sensory pain experienced, and reduce the emotional suffering with pain. Some patient groups in an Italian study also showed reduced medical utilization.

Following Donaldson's protocol, mentioned earlier, one can utilize muscle biofeedback to identify goals for an entire program of muscle rehabilitation, integrating relaxation skills with physical therapy. Donaldson uses biofeedback instruments to identify: (1) high patterns of standing muscle tension, which are probably present much of each day; (2) muscle asymmetry, that is, differences in the amount of tension on the left and right sides of the body; (3) co-activation of noninvolved muscles, which "join in" and tense along with the more appropriate muscles; and (4) failure to recover to a relaxed state after exertion. Then he prescribes stretching exercises to correct the postural imbalances and lengthen muscles and restore muscle fitness. The biofeedback instruments show whether the abnormal patterns improve with physical therapy. In addition, one can use the muscle biofeedback to guide the trainee to become more aware of the sensations they experience when the muscles are tensing and when they are relaxing. Awareness is only the beginning, the individual then works on reducing the activation of the sympathetic nervous system that causes the muscles to contract. This is difficult because individuals normally have very little, if any, control over their autonomic nervous system. Gaining control over muscle contractions is a trial and error process with the trainer guiding the trainee through the process and helping them to overcome obstacles to training as they occur.

Some individuals with fibromyalgia are able to learn to relax without the use of biofeedback. This is especially true for those whose fibromyalgia is of gradual onset when the pain is of mild severity. Some individuals find that relaxation tapes are helpful while others do not. When simple relaxation techniques do not provide relief, training by a therapist is suggested. Some therapists use a form of muscle relaxation developed by Edmund Jacobson[11] called progressive muscle relaxation (PMR), which is beneficial to those suffering from mild to moderately severe fibromyalgia. PMR involves working one's way systematically through each muscle group in the body. The emphasis is on awareness as much as control. The trainee tenses a muscle unit or group, and observes and feels the pattern of tension. While tensing, the trainee subjectively senses the control signal involved in tensing that muscle. The trainee now releases the tension in that muscle, "turns off the power," and allows the muscle to relax. The trainee sets aside any sense of effort or striving. Any effort to *make* the muscle relax will trigger new tension. After releasing the muscle, the trainee observes and comes to fine-tune an awareness and sensitivity for any residual tension. Over time, the trainee begins to spontaneously report more regularly recognizing states of tension and relaxation in everyday life. Donaldson and Sella[9] recommend using progressive muscle relaxation to reduce muscle resting tension levels, but with some caution, so as to avoid aggravating muscle imbalances and co-activations. The trainee may wish to introduce an element of gentleness—gently tensing muscles, while observing and feeling the tension that results.

Combining muscle biofeedback instruments with PMR allows one to assess and show the trainee how he or she is doing in relaxing muscles, reducing the number of noninvolved muscles "joining in" with appropriate muscles and balancing left–right patterns of muscle tension.

Balancing the Body: Heart Rhythm Training

A new form of biofeedback has emerged in the past decade, to restore balance in the body's autonomic nervous system.[12] Heart rhythm training, also called heart rate variability (HRV) biofeedback, is used to restore a coherent organized pattern in our autonomic nervous system, with positive benefit for many chronic medical problems.

The human heart beats at an ever-changing rate. The variability in heart rate is an adaptive quality in a healthy body. By variability I mean changes in the interval or distance between one beat of the heart and the next, as measured in milliseconds. This interval is highly variable within any given time period. High variability predicts better health, including better survival from a heart attack.[13] Low variability predicts poor health and greater risk of sudden death, especially death related to the cardiovascular system.

The body's autonomic nervous system (ANS) governs many of the body's internal functions, through natural pacemakers in the body. The sympathetic branch of the ANS activates or increases the heart's action, while the parasympathetic branch acts as a brake slowing the action of the heart. The vagus nerve plays a role in the parasympathetic braking action. The balance between this throttle and brake system produces an ongoing oscillation, an orderly increase and decrease in heart rate. Training in HRV biofeedback does not simply increase the power of either branch of the nervous system—parasympathetic or sympathetic—rather it exercises the balance between the two.

This physiology is relevant for fibromyalgia, because emerging research, conducted in the United States, Israel, Mexico, and elsewhere, is confirming that patients with fibromyalgia often have chronically over-activated sympathetic activity, under-active parasympathetic activity, decreased 24-hour heart rate variability, and elevated heart rates.[14,15,16] Similar findings have been reported for chronic fatigue syndrome, which overlaps with fibromyalgia.[17] Each of these physiological findings can be addressed and moderated by heart rate variability biofeedback.

In HRV biofeedback, the biofeedback practitioner begins by instructing the trainee to breathe slowly, smoothly, and evenly. Next, the trainee learns to set aside or release negative emotions and anxieties, and to cultivate warm, positive emotions. One might image cuddling a baby or holding the hand of a sick friend. The biofeedback instrument monitors both breath and heart rate, and soon, as the negative emotions fall away and breathing smoothes out, the computer screen will show two parallel sine waves—smooth hills and valleys representing breathing and heart rate. When anxiety and other influences lessen, breath becomes a dominant factor driving heart rate. With each inhalation, heart rate rises gently, and with each exhalation, heart rate gently drops. A special display, called a spectral analysis, will show a single peak frequency in heart rate activity, determined by the rate of breathing, and other influences on heart rate recede.

With practice, trainees are also able to increase the total variability in heart rate. One way to measure this variability is to measure the size of the swings from one's top heart rate to one's lowest heart rate, with each breath. Young athletic individuals may produce a swing, after training, of 20–50 beats/minute with each breath. Older individuals, especially those who lead sedentary lifestyles, will often show a swing of only 3–10 beats/minute. This loss of variability is a predictor of lessened physical vitality.

This very simple biofeedback procedure can be taught with relatively inexpensive biofeedback equipment. Case reports and recent research suggest that heart rate variability biofeedback can improve sleep in fibromyalgia, improve mood, and reduce pain.[18,19,20]

When an individual deliberately quiets the mind and body, this evokes what is called the biological *relaxation response*. The relaxation response erases the negative effects of stress on the human body. Breathing becomes slower and deeper, heart rate slows, muscles relax, and thinking becomes more relaxed. Practicing the relaxation response keeps human beings healthier, and induces greater calmness. Medical research shows that persons who practice relaxation don't catch colds and flu as often, have fewer accidents, and feel better in body and mind. Persons who practice relaxation regularly show calmer feelings, clearer thinking, and greater well-being.[21,22]

Many everyday activities can induce a mild relaxation response, including taking a walk along the beach, listening to quiet music, practicing a hobby, or working quietly in a garden. Identifying your own natural forms of relaxation, and giving them more place in your life, is a useful wellness strategy. However, individuals with moderate to severe fibromyalgia often need to learn relaxation techniques that can have a deeper effect on calming your body's tensions.

Earlier we discussed progressive muscle relaxation, muscle biofeedback, and heart rate variability training, all of which also produce some general relaxation. There are many other forms of relaxation training, including autogenic training, diaphragmatic breathing exercises, and a host of meditation techniques.[23,24]

Diaphragmatic Breathing

Paced, diaphragmatic breathing is an important tool in creating a relaxed state of body and mind, and is an element within many other relaxation and meditation strategies. The diaphragm is a dome-shaped muscle between the lungs and the abdominal cavity. Each time one inhales, the diaphragm contracts and flattens its curve, creating a vacuum into which the lungs can expand. As this happens the diaphragm pushes the abdominal muscles outward. The stomach of a baby visibly rises and falls as it breathes, and one can see this natural process in action. Many adults, however, because of tension, illness, or the desire to have a thin waist, resist this natural movement and have to relearn it.

Many therapists teach a variety of these relaxation techniques, and then use biofeedback instruments as well, to assess how well and how comprehensively the trainee is relaxing his or her body. Many individuals declare themselves relaxed, for example, yet continue to show elevated shoulder muscle tension, cold hands, or other indications of physiological stress.

Relaxation skills can moderate fibromyalgia pain, and often moderate other features of the disorder, such as sleep disorder, tender point sensitivity, and overall feelings of well-being. Buckelew et al. showed that relaxation, assisted by biofeedback training, raised the trainee's sense of self-efficacy—the confidence that he or she can do something to improve his or her condition.[25]

Relaxation is most effective when it is combined with other wellness-oriented skill education. Keel et al.[26] conducted a study showing that it is more effective to provide an integrated program that includes patient education, relaxation skills, exercise, and cognitive behavioral skills than to provide a single form of relaxation training in isolation. Buckelew et al.'s[25] study also compared relaxation alone to exercise, and to a combination group receiving both exercise and relaxation. Each group showed improvement, but the benefits lasted longer for the subjects receiving both relaxation and exercise. So whenever possible, individuals with fibromyalgia either should seek out an integrated program providing many self-regulation–oriented skills and activities or should construct their own program by enrolling in several classes and programs, such as yoga, exercise, and meditation skills.

Hypnosis and Self-Hypnosis

Can you form vivid visual images in your mind? Can you imagine biting a lemon, and find yourself puckering up and experiencing the bitterness? If so, you are probably a fairly good candidate for hypnosis, self-hypnosis, and imagery therapies.

Hypnosis is a very natural state of mind with several identifying characteristics. When in hypnosis, many individuals report an extraordinary quality of relaxation and an altered state of consciousness. Many hypnotic subjects show an unusual openness to the hypnotist's suggestions, and an ability to transform their everyday experiences of body, mind, and emotions. Most qualities that can be experienced in hypnosis by a hypnotist can also be accomplished, with learning and practice, through self-hypnosis.

One study provided 40 fibromyalgia patients with either hypnotherapy or traditional physical therapy.[27] The patients in the hypnotherapy group showed significantly better outcomes, with greater pain reduction, less fatigue on awakening, improved sleep patterns, and increased overall well-being. In addition, those patients treated with hypnotherapy showed a significant improvement in their overall levels of comfort. The authors concluded that hypnotherapy is effective in relieving the symptoms of fibromyalgia.

Balancing the Brain: Neurofeedback and Audio-Visual Entrainment

Neurofeedback

Neurofeedback is a fairly new therapy that uses an electroencephalograph (EEG) to measure brain electrical activity, and feeds back information on brain processes to the patient. Through feedback, the patient can learn to modify brain electrical patterns, just as he or she can tense or relax a muscle.[28] The primary goal of neurofeedback is to "normalize" brain activity—to modify brain rhythms so that they more closely resemble those of the healthy normal brain.

Neurofeedback is an effective therapeutic tool for many individuals with fibromyalgia; however, a lengthy course of treatment is often necessary. Patients may require anywhere from 10 to 50 sessions to achieve adequate and enduring changes in brain electrical activity. On the positive side, neurofeedback produces lasting changes in brain activity, which continue to be beneficial long after the treatment ceases. Unfortunately many insurance companies continue to label neurofeedback as expensive, and decline to reimburse the costs of neurofeedback treatment.

Audio-Visual Entrainment

Another promising new technology, called audio-visual entrainment (AVE), has been developed to shorten the process of normalizing brain rhythms. AVE uses light goggles and audio earphones to present flashing light and throbbing sound at programmed frequencies. The effects are more temporary than neurofeedback.

How Can You Benefit?

This chapter has reviewed a large number of mind–body therapies that offer help for those with fibromyalgia. One major advantage of the mind–body therapies is that they draw on the positive healing resources in the person, and do not share the many negative effects of pharmaceutical treatment.

Mind–body therapies can also be effectively combined with other interventions for fibromyalgia, including medication, nutritional supplements, acupuncture, and other alternative therapies.[29] As mentioned earlier, the most effective way to provide mind–body therapies is through a structured organized program that combines patient education, nutrition, exercises, and one or more mind–body therapies into a single group-based program. The group itself also becomes a part of the positive healing, because groups impart hope and model success for those beaten down by chronic conditions.[30] If a community lacks such an integrated program, then patients will benefit most by constructing their own multi-discipline program from the pieces that are available locally.

Mind–body therapies are not equally available in all communities. Most communities will include some therapists who have training in relaxation training skills, hypnosis, and general stress management. Most communities also include aqua therapy programs, usually in conjunction with hospital-based physical therapy programs. Most communities also have at least one yoga school. Even muscle biofeedback is relatively available, at least in any community with a university or hospital-based health center. Therapists with training in the use of neurofeedback, audio-visual entrainment, and heart rate variability biofeedback are less available.

Those searching for mind–body therapists also face a bewildering array of professional credentials. How is one to determine a therapist's level of competence? Patients should always ask very specific questions about the professional's degree, license, certification, and training in their specialty area. Most mind–body therapies are more effective when provided by licensed health care professionals who have completed a structured program of professional training with additional training in their specialty area. Any psychologist or physician, for example, may legally purchase biofeedback equipment and offer biofeedback services. Reputable biofeedback therapists, however, attend biofeedback training workshops regularly, and seek certification. It is often helpful for patients to check with their own open-minded physician about the competence of mind–body therapists in the community.

The best online resource for finding competent biofeedback and neurofeedback therapists is the Biofeedback Certification Institute of America, which maintains a list of certified practitioners on its web site (www.bcia.org).

Finally, do not lose hope! Fibromyalgia is a real medical condition that causes enormous suffering. However, it is not life-threatening, and promising therapies are now emerging regularly. There is no need to give in to a lifetime of disability. It is possible to begin with simple steps toward wellness—improving sleep quality, getting more physical exercise, and making better nutritional choices. If necessary, seek out the available mind–body therapists in your community, and begin the slow steady path of rehabilitation and recovery.

Resources

Burke A. *Self Hypnosis De-mystified: New Tools for Deep and Lasting Trans-formation.* Berkeley, CA: Crossing Press; 2004.

Caprio F, Berger J, Miller C. *Healing Yourself with Self-Hypnosis.* Upper Saddle River, NJ: Prentice Hall Press; 1998.

Davis M, Eshelman ER, McKay M. (2000). *Relaxation and Stress Reduction Workbook.* Oakland, CA: New Harbinger Workbooks; 2000.

Fransen J, Russell IJ. *The Fibromyalgia Help Book: Practical Guide to Living Better with Fibromyalgia.* St. Paul, MI: Smith House Press; 1996.

Hauri P, Jarman M, Linde S. *No More Sleepless Nights Workbook.* New York, NY: Wiley; 2001.

Moss D, McGrady A, Davies T, Wickramasekera I, eds. *Handboook of Mind–Body Medicine in Primary Care.* Thousand Oaks, CA: Sage Publications; 2003.

References

1. Quintner J. Fibromyalgia: The Copenhagen Declaration. *Lancet.* 1992;340(8827):1103.
2. Donaldson CCS, Sella GE, Mueller HH. Fibromyalgia: a retrospective study of 252 consecutive referrals. *Can J Clin Med.* 1998;5(6):116-127.
3. Perlis ML, Giles DE, Bootzin RR, et al. Alpha sleep and information processing, perception of sleep, pain and arousability in fibromyalgia. *Int J Neurosci.* 1997;80(3-4):265-280.

4. Cohen H, Neumann L, Shore M, et al. Autonomic dysfunction in patients with fibromyalgia: application of power spectral analysis of heart rate variability. *Semin Arthritis Rheum.* 2000:29(4);197-199.

5. Martinez-Lavin M, Hermosillo AG, Rosas M, Soto ME. Circadian studies of autonomic nervous balance in patients with fibromyalgia: a heart rate variability analysis. *Arthritis Rheum.* 1998;41(11):1966-1971.

6. Vaeroy H. Altered sympathetic nervous system response in patients with fibromyalgia. *J Rheum.* 1989;16(11): 1460-1465.

7. Drexler AR, Mur EJ, Gunther VC. Efficacy of an EMG-biofeedback therapy in fibromyalgia patients. A comparative study of patients with and without abnormality in (MMPI) psychological scales. *Clin Exp Rheum.* 2002;20(5):677-682.

8. Mur E, Drexler A, Gruber J, Hartig F, Gunther V. Electromyography biofeedback therapy in fibromyalgia. *Wiener medizinische Wochenschrift.* 1999;149(19-20):561-563.

9. Donaldson CCS, Sella G. Fibromyalgia. In: Moss D, McGrady A, Davies T, Wickramasekera I, eds. *Handbook of Mind–Body Medicine for Primary Care.* Thousand Oaks, CA: Sage; 2003:323-332.

10. Gilbert C, Moss D. Biofeedback. In: Moss D, McGrady A, Davies T, Wickramasekera I, eds. *Handbook of Mind–Body Medicine for Primary Care.* Thousand Oaks, CA: Sage; 2003:109-122.

11. Jacobson E. *Progressive Relaxation.* Chicago, IL: University of Chicago Press; 1938.

12. Moss D. Heart rate variability and biofeedback. *Psychophysiology Today: The Magazine for Mind–Body Medicine.* 2004;1:4-11. Available at: http://www.bfe.org/library.html. Accessed November 1, 2006.

13. DelPozo J, Gevirtz RN, Scher B, Guarneri E. Biofeedback treatment increases heart rate variability in patients with known coronary artery disease. *Am Heart J.* 2004;147(3):E11.

14. Cohen H, Neumann L, Shore M, Amir M, Cassuto Y, Buskila D. Autonomic dysfunction in patients with fibromyalgia: application of power spectral analysis of heart rate variability. *Semin Arthritis Rheum.* 2000;29(4):197-199.

15. Martinez-Lavin M, Hermosillo AG, Rosas M, Soto ME. Circadian studies of autonomic nervous balance in patients with fibromyalgia: a heart rate variability analysis. *Arthritis Rheum.* 1998;41(11):1966-1971.

16. Raj SR, Brouillard D, Simpson CS, Hopman WM, Abdollah H. Dysautonomia among patients with fibromyalgia: a noninvasive assessment. *J Rheum.* 2000;27(11):2660-2665.

17. Sisto SA, Tapp W, Drastal S, et al. Vagal tone is reduced during paced breathing in patients with the chronic fatigue syndrome. *Clin Auton Res.* 1995;5(3):139-143.

18. Gevirtz RN. The promise of HRV biofeedback: some preliminary results and speculations. *Biofeedback.* 2003;31(3):18-19.

19. Gevirtz RN. Resonant frequency training to restore homeostasis for treatment of psychophysiological disorders. *Biofeedback.* 2000;27:7-9.

20. Radvanski D, Vaschillo EG, Vaschillo B, Hassett AL, Lehrer PM, Sigal L. Heart rate variability biofeedback for fibromyalgia treatment. Paper presented at: Annual Meeting of the Association for Applied Psychophysiology and Biofeedback; April, 2004; Austin, TX.

21. Gruzelier J. (2002). A review of the impact of hypnosis, relaxation, guided imagery and individual differences on aspects of immunity and health. *Stress.* 2002;5(2):147-163.

22. Lehrer PM, Woolfolk RL, eds. *Principles and Practice of Stress Management.* 2nd ed. New York, NY: Guilford Press; 1993.

23. Davis M, Eshelman ER, McKay M. *Relaxation and Stress Reduction Workbook.* Oakland, CA: New Harbinger Workbooks; 2000.

24. Lehrer PM, Carrington P. Relaxation, autogenic training, and meditation. In: Moss D, Wickramasekera I, McGrady A, Davies T, eds. *Handbook of Mind–Body Medicine in Primary Care.* Thousand Oaks, CA: Sage; 2003:137-149.

25. Buckelew SP, Conway R, Parker J, et al. Biofeedback/relaxation training and exercise interventions for fibromyalgia: a prospective trial. *Arthritis Care Res.* 1998;11(3):196-209.

26. Keel PJ, Bodoky C, Gerhard U, Muller W. (1998). Comparison of integrated group therapy and group relaxation training for fibromyalgia. *Clin J Pain.* 1998;14(3):232-238.

27. Haanen HC, Hoenderdos HT, van Romunde LK, et al. (1991). Controlled trial of hypnotherapy in the treatment of refractory fibromyalgia. *J Rheum.* 1991;18(1):72-75.

28. LaVaque T. Neurofeedback, neurotherapy, and quantitative EEG. In: Moss D, McGrady A, Davies T, Wickramasekera I, eds. *Handbook of Mind–Body Medicine for Primary Care.* Thousand Oaks, CA: Sage; 2003:123-135.

29. Moss D, McGrady A, Davies T, Wickramasekera I, eds. *Handbook of Mind–Body Medicine in Primary Care.* Thousand Oaks, CA: Sage; 2003.

30. Gordon JS, Moss D. (2003). Manifesto for a new medicine. *Biofeedback.* 2003;31(3):8-11, 19.

Did You Get the License Number of the Truck That Hit Me?

Jenny Melkvik

*Jenny recently retired from teaching but continues to
tutor many former math students. She enjoys spending
time with her parents and family and traveling,
and appreciates her many blessings.*

— •◆• —

We think of fibromyalgia as something that happens to *other* people, people we don't even know. How different it seems when it happens to you. It did happen to me.

Why should you care to hear about my case? Indeed, every case of fibromyalgia is unique. And the onset of this disease is unique in each patient. Nonetheless, in the stories of individual patients certain patterns emerge, or at least suggest themselves. For example, the onset of fibromyalgia often follows some serious injury or illness. Are some people genetically predisposed to fibromyalgia so that they fall prey to it after such an injury or illness? Another common theme is that, because there are so many mysterious symptoms and because the pain occurs in so many places, fibromyalgia is often misdiagnosed or regarded as "all in the patient's head." One thing is for sure, fibromyalgia always has a tremendous impact on the patient's life. Therefore, in this chapter, I'm going to tell you about fibromyalgia from a patient's perspective, to give you an idea of what the journey to proper treatment and beyond is like.

I don't know whether it began with my normal fall allergies or a cold, but on October 19, 1999, I was diagnosed with bronchitis. After two sets of antibiotics failing, my principal forcing me to stay home from my teaching job, and my mother telling me I should go to the emergency room, I finally listened. I had really done it this time—bilateral pneumonia with a fever of more than 105. I was hospitalized for a week until the intravenous antibiotics knocked down the infection.

I survived. However, my doctor warned me that my immune system was damaged and that it would be a year before it was functioning again and capable of protecting me from disease. I was out of the classroom for a month, checking in with my doctor weekly. Each time he told me that teaching is the worst kind of work after such a serious illness, because kids crowded into schools are the perfect breeding ground for every type of germ.

I was back in school two days . . . and back to the doctor on the third. You guessed it: I caught something from the kids. My doctor wanted me back in the hospital, but I didn't want to go and promised to take a couple more days off to rest before returning to work again.

Thanksgiving week gave me more time to rest. The following week I saw the doctor again, and things were as good as could be expected for someone recovering from double pneumonia. Then in February 2000 the migraines hit hard. Light hurt my eyes, I felt nauseous, and the pain was excruciating. A neurologist tried Imitrex, but it left me feeling very strange. An anticonvulsant, Depakote, finally eliminated the migraines. I took it for six months before the doctor weaned me off.

I don't exactly remember when the rest of my symptoms started. But I do remember that in January 2002 I went to my primary-care physician to get all my aches and pains checked out before returning to school after the holidays. I remember telling her that I had been working out and that my muscles and joints ached, so I had eased up. I had already been diagnosed with Raynaud's syndrome, a central nervous system disorder in which the blood stops flowing to the extremities whenever you feel cold. I told her that it seemed worse because my fingers and hands were often numb. She decided to send me back to the neurologist for an EMG (a nerve conduction test) to have the numbness checked out.

The neurologist did an EMG, which suggested carpal tunnel syndrome in both wrists. This diagnosis made no sense and frustrated me. I went to the doctor because I was in pain, great pain all over, and came out with a diagnosis of carpal tunnel? A teacher? Teachers don't get carpal tunnel! Now what?

He prescribed braces for both wrists, advising that I wear them 24 hours a day, but if that didn't work out for me, I could wear them only while sleeping. This doctor didn't seem to care at all about my pain.

One month later, I was in too much pain to still be angry, so I went back to my primary-care physician. I told her I wasn't sleeping now, on top of it all. Though I fell asleep easily, because I was always exhausted, a few hours later I awoke in intense pain. I'd eventually fall back to sleep, only to awake in pain again—and I repeated this cycle throughout the night, night after night. Sometimes I awoke feeling like I hadn't slept at all. Imagine having trouble sleeping and knocking yourself in the head with braces on both wrists!

My physician and I talked. She asked me many questions, poking my body in specific places—near the neck, elbows, hips, knees, and several other places. It was as if she knew right where to press to hurt me! She kept pausing to refer to a book on the counter behind her and then asking me more questions. It seemed to me that she was doing that for an awfully long time. While I lay there thinking, I remembered that my mother had read in her nursing journal about a disease called fibromyalgia. Mom thought my symptoms sounded just like the symptoms described in the article. She had told me that I should ask my doctor to rule out fibromyalgia. At the very moment I was remembering this, the doctor announced, "I think you have fibromyalgia."

From the look on her face, I could tell this was serious, but I didn't know what fibromyalgia was. She sat down and told me many things, while I went into shock and didn't hear much. The things I do remember hearing that day are *chronic . . . no cure . . . you will have it forever . . . a lot of doctors don't believe it's a real disease . . . pain all over your body . . . problems sleeping . . . difficult to diagnose and treat.* We discussed my current pain levels and sleeping problems. She prescribed sleep medication and told me to try Tylenol for the pain. She would have preferred ibuprofen, but since I have a history of esophageal spasms, my throat and stomach are too sensitive to take it.

True to my nature as a teacher, I was now on a frantic search to find out everything there was to know about fibromyalgia. And so was my mother, mainly because she is my mother, but also because she is a retired nurse. Within two weeks we found and attended a seminar on fibromyalgia. The seminar provided more information about fibromyalgia, and gave me ideas on how to reduce the pain. Unfortunately, this seminar's purpose was mainly to sell a vitamin supplement program touting miraculous cures for fibromyalgia. I had already spent enough money on several vitamin supplement programs with no improvement, so I was not interested in going in that direction again.

A week later, I was back at the doctor. Tylenol doesn't touch this kind of pain, and my blood pressure was too high—pain causes it to rise. So she added blood pressure pills to my growing list of medications.

In May 2002, I was desperate for greater relief. I read that massage is very helpful. My friend is a massage therapist. Being a dear friend, he read up on fibromyalgia and was ready for me! Unfortunately, he cared so much that he gave me a wonderfully deep massage, found every tender point on my body, and the next day I was in so much pain I could barely move.

During the next few months, I underwent ankle-implant surgery, and the fibromyalgia went from one flare-up to another. I couldn't tell what was causing my pain—the injury, the swelling, the incision, or the fibromyalgia itself. My primary-care physician decided she could no longer treat the pain, because it was more than could be handled by diet, exercise, Tylenol, and gentle sleep medications. She referred me to a pain management clinic. I didn't know there were doctors whose whole practice is to help patients manage pain, but I sure am glad there are.

When I met my pain management doctor in October 2002, he was interested in what my pain level was at that moment, how intense it got, what the monthly average was, and how well I was sleeping. I left that day with prescriptions for pain and sleep aids, knowing I had a doctor who would listen and help me.

You might think that someone going through all of this might be going crazy. Well, I'm not saying I wasn't. The doctors at the pain clinic soon referred me to a psychologist who works with fibromyalgia patients and specializes in treating people living in chronic pain. It was wonderful to talk to someone who had studied fibromyalgia. He could finish my sentences about the pain. His face showed not only that he was listening, but that he really cared. He helped me manage the pain and find ways to relax. Equally important, he taught me ways to say "No." All my life, I've tried to do everything for everyone all the time. It has been hard for me to accept that I can no longer do that, and it's been hard for others to understand. I see this wonderful psychologist regularly.

Long trips in the car are difficult for me. My pain clinic doctor suggested I try a TENS unit. Through pads attached to your body at points of pain, it sends electrical impulses to the muscles, breaking the pain cycle. It feels a little like a massage, and it helps. I use this off and on for long road trips.

I go to the pain clinic religiously each month. We noticed a pattern with my pain. Most of it was in my lower back. My pain doctor had been giving me injections into the base of the spine, which gave me some relief. In March 2004, he sent me for an MRI, which indicated severe disc problems. We agreed that surgery should be a last resort.

Then in November 2004, I awoke one morning with the front of my left thigh completely numb and the side on fire. Time for the last resort. I was referred to an orthopedic back surgeon who could see me on January 19, 2005!

As my pain had been increasing over the years, my dosage of Vicodin had been gradually increased as well. Over time, a Duragesic pain patch was added to my list of medications, replacing the Vicodin. This pain patch is something you can't just start with—you must slowly work up to it. I started with a 25 mcg/hour patch. I still had much breakthrough pain, so it was adjusted up to 50 mcg/hour. I now wear a 75 mcg/hour patch, and even with this dosage I have breakthrough pain. To receive these stronger medications, I agreed to an opioid contract that spelled out my responsibilities, which I followed to the letter.

On May 20, 2005, I had spinal fusion surgery. That summer I was exhausted all the time. I slept more than 11 hours a night and sometimes took a nap or two during the day. The numbness on the top of my thigh and the burning-poker pain on the side were gone, but I still had the fibromyalgia pain I'd had before the surgery. As the new school year approached, I got more and more worried that I would not be able to return to work. I was too exhausted and in too much pain.

During the first weeks of August, I visited my surgeon, my pain clinic doctors, and my psychologist looking for help. I love teaching more than just about anything! Last year my principal—bless her heart—got permission for me to have first-hour planning so I could use it for physical therapy or extra rest. I knew she would do that again for me, but I did not think it would be enough. I decided to attempt this with a doctor's note saying that I would need to be absent when I was feeling exhausted. That agreement did not turn out to be enough. The next doctor's note forced me to take off every Wednesday. When that was not enough, I decided to take an unpaid leave of absence for the rest of the school year. This gave me a lot of time to think, and I made the hardest decision of my life. I decided to take a disability retirement.

The stress of not hearing the alarm has eased since I retired, but it is still very difficult for me to wake up in the morning. I still don't have the energy to do all the things that I want. I feel like I am always playing "catch up." I work much slower due to the pain and the "brain fog" of fibromyalgia. I used to love the feeling of having all important tasks completed. Now, when I literally don't have the time, strength, or energy to do them I don't let it bother me. Many people don't understand, so I try to get close to people who do understand. My family and I need to adjust our thinking from what I once could do to what I can do now. I am not the same person I was before fibromyalgia, but I still have a lot to give.

My life's focus has changed. Each day I need to count my blessings, look for people who I can help, find ways to educate people about fibromyalgia, and "squeeze in" my almost daily doctor appointments, tests, and physical therapy. My physical therapist specializes in fibromyalgia. He uses an almost entirely hands-on massage treatment that does not cause me more pain. This has been a tremendous benefit to me. In addition, my current medications are helping.

Looking back, my improvements have been thanks to the combined efforts of my physicians, therapists, and all the supportive people who have come into my life.

Resources

Web Sites

American Academy of Craniofacial Pain
520 West Pipeline Road
Hurst, TX 76053
www.aacfp.org

American Academy of Medical Acupuncture
4929 Wilshire Boulevard
Suite 428
Los Angeles, CA 90010
(323) 937-5514
www.medicalacupuncture.org

American Academy of Pain Medicine
13947 Mono Way #A
Sonora, CA 95370
(209) 533-9744
www.painmed.org

American Academy of Physical Medicine and Rehabilitation
One IBM Plaza, Suite 2500
Chicago, IL 60611
(312) 464-9700
www.aapmr.org

American Academy of Sleep Medicine
One Westbrook Corporate Center, Suite 920
Westchester, IL 60154
www.aasmnet.org

American Botanical Council
www.herbalgram.org

American Chronic Pain Association
P.O. Box 850
Rocklin, CA 95677
(800) 533-3231
www.theacpa.org

American College of Rheumatology
1800 Century Place, Suite 250
Atlanta, GA 30345-4300
(404) 633-3777
www.rheumatology.org

American Fibromyalgia Syndrome Association
6380 E. Tanque Verde, Suite D
Tucson, AZ 85715
(520) 733-1570
www.afsafund.org

American Massage Therapy Association
820 Davis Street
Evanston, IL 60201
(847) 864-0123
www.amtamassage.org

American Optometric Association
www.aoa.org

American Pain Foundation
201 N. Charles Street, Suite 710
Baltimore, MD 21201-4111
www.painfoundation.org

American Pain Society
4700 W. Lake Avenue
Glenview, IL 60025
(847) 375-4715
www.ampainsoc.org

American Physical Therapy Association
1111 N. Fairfax St.
Alexandria, VA 22314
(800) 999-2782
www.apta.org

Aquatic Resources Network
3500 E. Vicksburg Lane, #250
Portsmouth, NH 55447
www.aquaticnet.com

Arthritis Foundation
P.O. Box 7669
Atlanta, GA 30357-0669
(800) 687-2277
www.arthritis.org

Association for Applied Psychophysiology and Biofeedback
10200 W. 44th Avenue, Suite 304
Wheat Ridge, CO 80033-2840
(303) 422-8436
www.aapb.org

Biofeedback Certification Institute of America
10200 W. 44th Avenue, Suite 310
Wheat Ridge, CO 80033-2840
(866) 908-8713
www.bcia.org

Centers for Disease Control and Prevention
1600 Clifton Rd.
Atlanta, GA 30333
(800) 311-3435
www.cdc.gov

Chronic Pain and Fatigue Research Center
www.med.umich.edu/painresearch

Division of Rheumatology at the University of Michigan
www.med.umich.edu/intmed/rheumatology

Fibromyalgia Network
6380 E. Tanque Verde, Suite D
Tucson, AZ 85715
(520) 290-5508
www.fmnetnews.com

Food and Drug Administration
www.fda.gov

Helping Our Pain and Exhaustion
23915 Forest Park
Novi, MI 48374
(248) 344-0896
www.hffcf.org

International Association for Chronic Fatigue Syndrome
27 N. Wacker Drive, Suite 416
Chicago, IL 60606
www.aacfs.org

Job Accommodation Network
www.jan.wvu.edu/media/Fibro.html

Massage Finder Information
http://www.massagetherapy.com/home/index.php

Medline Plus
www.nlm.nih.gov/medlineplus/fibromyalgia.html

Medline Plus Drug Information Website
http://www.nlm.nih.gov/medlineplus/druginformation.html

National Center for Complementary and Alternative Medicine
NCCAM Clearinghouse
P.O. Box 7923
Gaithersburg, MD 20898
(888) 644-6226
www.nccam.nih.gov

National Fibromyalgia Association
2200 N. Glassel Street, Suite A
Orange, CA 92865
(714) 921-0150
www.fmaware.org

National Fibromyalgia Partnership
www.fmpartnership.org

National Headache Foundation
820 N. Orleans, Suite 217
Chicago, IL 60610
(888) NHF-5552
www.headaches.org

National Women's Health Resource Center
157 Broad Street, Suite 315
Red Bank, NJ 07701
(877) 986-9742
www.healthywomen.org

NIH Office of Dietary Supplements
http://ods.od.nih.gov

Partnership for Prescription Assistance
www.pparx.org

Restless Legs Syndrome Foundation
304 Glenwood Avenue
Raleigh, NC 27603-1455
www.rls.org

Thyroid Foundation of America
One Longfellow Place, Suite 1518
Boston, MA 02114
(800) 832-8321
www.allthyroid.org

The TMJ Association
P.O. Box 27660
Milwaukee, WI 53226
(262) 432-0350
www.tmj.org

USDA Nutrient Data Laboratory
www.nal.usda.gov/fnic/foodcomp/search

Vulvar Pain Foundation
203 North Main Street, Suite 203
Graham, NC 27253
(336) 226-0704
www.vulvarpainfoundation.org

Womenshealth.gov
http://www.4woman.gov/

Magazines

Fibromyalgia AWARE Magazine
www.FMaware.org/magazine.html

Massage Magazine
www.massagemag.com

Yoga Journal
www.yogajournal.com

Medical Journals

Journal of Musculoskeletal Pain
www.haworthpress.com

DVD's

Living With Fibromyalgia DVD: A journey of hope and under-standing
http://www.livingwithfm.com/order_dvd.html

Yoga for Healing, deluxe DVD edition, includes a total of 3 hours of yoga arranged in seven graded 10–30-minute practices, ranging from very gentle yoga that can be done on a bed or chair, through moderately challenging practices for people whose fibromyalgia is in remission.
www.downwarddogproductions.net

Web site: http://sharonostalecki.com

"Best of Aware" (Volume 1–5) CD. Fibromyalgia AWARE maga-zine: www.fmaware.org.

Glossary

Acetaminophen: The generic name for Tylenol.

ACTH: Adrenocorticotropic hormone, is a pituitary hormone that stimulates the secretion of glucocorticoids (such as cortisol) from the adrenal cortex.

Acupuncture: The practice of piercing specific sites on the body, called pathways or meridians, with thin needles in an attempt to relieve pain associated with some chronic disorders.

Acute: Condition of short duration that starts quickly and has severe symptoms.

ADHD: Attention deficit hyperactivity disorder.

Adjuvant therapies: Drugs that augment the effects of analgesics. They include antidepressants and anticonvulsants.

Adrenal insufficiency: A condition in which the body produces too little cortisol and/or aldosterone.

Aerobic exercise: Physical exercise that increases the work of the heart and lungs; examples are running, jogging, swimming, and dancing.

Allodynia: An altered sensation in which normally nonpainful events are felt as pain.

Alternative medicine: A broad category of treatment systems (e.g., chiropractic, herbal medicine, acupuncture, homeopathy, naturopathy, and spiritual devotions). Alternative medicine is also referred to as "complementary medicine." The designation "alternative medicine" is not equivalent to holistic medicine, a narrower term.

Anaerobic: Without oxygen.

Analgesic: A medication or agent that reduces pain.

Anecdotal: Evidence based on reports of specific individual cases rather than controlled, clinical studies.

Anticonvulsants: Drugs given to prevent seizures.

Autonomic nervous system: System of the brain that controls key bodily functions not under conscious control, such as heartbeat, breathing, and sweating. The autonomic nervous system has two divisions: the sympathetic nervous system accelerates heart rate, constricts blood vessels, and raises blood pressure; the parasympathetic nervous system slows heart rate, increases intestinal and gland activity, and relaxes sphincter muscles.

bid: Medication taken twice a day.

Biofeedback: The use of electronic instruments to measure muscle tension in any muscle group.

Carbohydrates: One of the three main classes of food and a source of energy. Carbohydrates are the sugars and starches found in breads, cereals, fruits, and vegetables. During digestion, carbo-hydrates are changed into a simple sugar called glucose.

Central nervous system: The brain and spinal cord.

Central sensitization: A malfunction in the brain pain recognition centers that causes people with fibromyalgia to experience pain instead of normal sensations.

Cervical region: The upper spine (neck) area of the vertebral column.

Chronic: A disease showing little changes or of slow progression; the opposite of acute.

Chronic fatigue syndrome: A condition of excessive fatigue, cognitive impairment, and other varied symptoms. Classified by the World Health Organization (WHO) as a disease of the nervous system, it is of unknown etiology and may last months or years, causing severe disability.

Circadian rhythm: A metabolic or behavior pattern that repeats in cycles of about every 24 hours.

Cognitive-behavioral therapy (CBT): A type of psychotherapy in which the therapist teaches the patient to restructure his or her cognitive beliefs, (i.e., thought patterns) and hence, behavior.

Complementary and alternative medicine (CAM): A group of diverse medical and health care systems, practices, and products that are not presently considered to be part of conventional medicine.

Compounding pharmacy: A facility that both makes and sells prescription drugs. A compounding pharmacy can often prepare drug formulas that are specially tailored to patients: for example, liquid versions of medications normally available only in pill form, for patients who cannot swallow pills.

Condyle: The joint portion of the lower jaw.

Costochondritis: Inflammation at the junction of a rib and its cartilage.

Craniosacral therapy: A gentle form of manipulation. Craniosacral therapists manipulate the craniosacral system, which includes the soft tissue and bones of the head (cranium), the spine down to its tail end (the sacral area), and the pelvis. They also work with the membranes that surround these bones and the cerebrospinal fluid that bathes the brain and spinal cord.

Degenerative joint disease: Osteoarthritis or rheumatoid arthritis.

Dolorimeter: A device for quantifying the threshold of pain.

Dry eye disease: Decreased tear production or increased tear film evaporation.

Elimination diet: A diet in which certain foods are temporarily discontinued from the diet to rule out the cause of allergy symptoms.

Endorphins: Any of a group of proteins with potent analgesic properties that occur naturally in the brain.

Essential fatty acids: Fatty acids that the body cannot manufacture, so it must obtain them from the diet. Examples are linolenic acid and linoleic acid, which are both found in evening primrose oil and flax seed oil. They are considered essential to good health.

Fascia: A fibrous membrane covering, supporting, and separating muscle and some organs of the body. Also known as soft tissue.

Feldenkrais: A system of bodywork developed by physicist Moshe Feldenkrais, to improve posture, movement, and breathing. Feldenkrais teaches recognizing and breaking improper habits of movement.

Fibro-fog: The cognitive dysfunction experienced by many fibromyalgia patients.

Fibromyalgia: A chronic disorder characterized by widespread musculoskeletal pain, fatigue, and multiple tender points that occur in precise, localized areas, particularly in the neck, spine, shoulders, and hips. It also may cause sleep disturbances, morning stiffness, irritable bowel syndrome, anxiety, and other symptoms.

Flexibility: The ability of muscle to relax and yield to stretch forces.

Functional capacity evaluation (FCE): A systematic process of assessing an individual's physical capacities and functional abilities.

Functional gastrointestinal disorders: Gastrointestinal disorders for which no biological disease process underlies the symptoms.

Gait: The way in which a person walks.

Ganglia: A mass of nerve tissue or a group of nerve cell bodies.

Ghrelin: A hormone that signals the body to eat and store fat.

Glucagon: A hormone that blocks the effects of insulin.

Glucose: The chief source of energy for living organisms.

Gluten: A protein group found in wheat and other flours that forms the structure of bread dough.

Glycemic index: A measure of how rapidly glucose from various forms of carbohydrates are digested and then absorbed into the blood circulation. Low glycemic index foods, limit the rush of blood glucose after a meal.

Graves' disease: Hyperthyroidism.

High-density lipoprotein (HDL): One of the classes of lipoproteins that carry cholesterol in the blood. HDL is considered to be beneficial because it removes excess cholesterol and disposes of it. Hence, HDL cholesterol is often termed "good" cholesterol.

Holistic medicine: Healing traditions that promote the protection and restoration of health through theories reputedly based on the body's natural ability to heal itself and by understanding the various ways body components affect each other and are influenced by the environment.

Hypermobile: Abnormally flexible.

Hyperpathia: Abnormally severe pain from a stimulus that normally is slightly painful.

Hyperthyroidism: Excessive functionality of the thyroid gland marked by increased metabolic rate, enlargement of the thyroid gland, rapid heart rate, high blood pressure, and various secondary symptoms.

Hypoglycemia: An abnormally low level of glucose in the blood.

Hypothyroidism: Underactivity of the thyroid gland, causing tiredness, cramps, a slowed heart rate, and possibly weight gain.

Hypoxic: Deficient in oxygen.

Immune system: The body system that protects the body against invading organisms and infections.

Initiating factors: Factors that cause the onset of myofascial pain.

Insomnia: Inadequate quality or quantity of sleep, with difficulty initiating or maintaining sleep.

Irritable bowel syndrome: A chronic functional gastrointestinal disorder primarily characterized by abdominal pain and disturbed bowel functioning (diarrhea and/or constipation). It is present in 33–77% of individuals with fibromyalgia.

Ischemia: Lack of blood flow to a body part, often caused by constriction or obstruction of a blood vessel.

Joint: The point of connection between two bones or elements of a skeleton (especially if the articulation allows motion).

Journaling: The process of recording information about your daily life.

Leptin: An appetite-suppressing hormone.

Ligament: A tough band of tissue connecting the articular extremities of bones or supporting an organ in place.

Low-density lipoprotein (LDL): The major cholesterol carrier in the blood. If there is too much LDL circulating in the blood, the cholesterol may be deposited in artery walls, contributing to atherosclerosis. It is sometimes called "bad" cholesterol.

Lumbar region: Pertaining to the lower back.

Lymph node: A rounded mass of lymphatic tissue that is surrounded by a capsule of connective tissue. Also known as a lymph gland. Lymph nodes are spread out along lymphatic vessels and they contain many lymphocytes, which filter the lymphatic fluid (lymph).

MAOs (monoamine oxidase): Any of a chemically similar group of drugs used primarily in the treatment of depression.

Massage therapy: Manipulation of tissues (as by rubbing, kneading, or tapping) with the hand or an instrument for therapeutic purposes.

Melatonin: Pineal hormone (a hormone secreted from the pineal gland) secreted primarily during the hours of darkness.

Meridians: The pathways of positive and negative energy power in the body.

Minerals: Organic substances needed in the diet in small amounts to help regulate body function.

MRI (magnetic resonance imaging): A noninvasive, non–X-ray diagnostic technique based on the magnetic fields of hydrogen atoms in the body. MRI provides computer-generated images of the body's internal tissues and organs.

Multidisciplinary approach: Approach that uses many experts from different disciplines working together as a team to manage and control the symptoms of fibromyalgia.

Muscle: A body tissue consisting of long cells that contract when stimulated and produce motion.

Myofascial pain: Pain and tenderness in the muscles and adjacent fibrous tissues (fascia).

Nerve blocks: Injections to treat or alleviate pain in a region by delivering medication to the nerve(s), which blocks the flow of pain signals.

Neurotransmitters: Chemicals in the brain, such as acetylcholine, serotonin, and norepinephrine, that facilitate communication between nerve cells (neurons).

Norepinephrine: A neurotransmitter found mainly in areas of the brain that are involved in governing autonomic nervous system activity, especially blood pressure and heart rate.

NREM (non-rapid eye movement): A recurring sleep state during which rapid eye movements do not occur and dreaming does not occur; accounts for about 75% of normal sleep time.

NSAIDs (nonsteroidal anti-inflammatory drugs): Drugs that act against inflammation, reduce fever, relieve muscle pain, and prevent blood clots.

Nutrition: The process by which an individual takes in and utilizes food material.

Nutritional therapy: Using food and supplements to encourage the body's natural healing.

Occlusal splint: A night guard for the mouth or orthotic appliance.

Opiates: Narcotics prepared or derived from opium.

Opioids: Synthetic narcotics that resemble opiates in action but that are not derived from opium.

Orthotic: Orthopedic appliance or apparatus used to support, align, prevent, or correct deformities or to improve the function of movable parts of the body.

Orthotist: A skilled professional who fabricates orthotic devices that are prescribed by a physician.

Palpate: To touch or feel.

Perpetuating factors: Factors that interfere with healing or enhance the progression of myofascial pain.

Physiatrist: A physician who specializes in physical medicine and rehabilitation.

Physical therapy: The treatment consisting of exercising specific parts of the body such as the legs, arms, hands, or neck in an effort to strengthen, regain range of motion, relearn movement, and/or rehabilitate the musculoskeletal system to improve function.

Polysomnography: A technical term for a sleep study that involves recording brain waves for assessing the quality of sleep and airflow at the nose and mouth.

Predisposing factors: Factors that increase the risk of myofascial pain.

Pronation: Rotation of the foot inward, when walking.

Protein: Complex molecules composed of amino acids that are essential to an organism structure and function. Meats, eggs and dairy products are significant sources of protein; however you can also get protein from a variety of grains, legumes, nuts and seeds. Proteins are the "building blocks" of the human body.

Psychiatrist: A medical doctor who specializes in the treatment and prevention of mental and emotional disorders.

Psychologist: A specialist who can talk with patients and their families about emotional and personal matters, and can help them make decisions.

q4h: Medication taken every 4 hours.

q12h: Medication taken every 12 hours.

qd: Medication taken every day.

Qi: Energy flow.

qid: Medication taken 4 times a day.

Raynaud's syndrome: Discoloration of the fingers or toes due to emotion or cold in a characteristic pattern over time: white, blue, and red.

RDA: Recommendations for daily intake of specific nutrients for groups of healthy individuals set by the Food and Nutrition Board of the National Research Council of the National Academy of Science.

Reactive hypoglycemia: Reactive hypoglycemia is a medical term describing recurrent episodes of hypoglycemia occurring 2–4 hours after a high carbohydrate meal (or oral glucose load). It is thought to represent a consequence of excessive insulin release triggered by the carbohydrate meal but continuing past the digestion and disposal of the glucose derived from the meal.

Referred pain: Pain from a malfunctioning or diseased area of the body that is perceived in another area, often far from the origin.

REM (rapid eye movement): A light sleep when dreams occur and the eyes move rapidly back and forth.

Rheumatoid arthritis (RA): A chronic disease characterized by stiffness and inflammation of the joints, loss of mobility, weakness, and deformity.

ROM: Range of motion. The amount of movement (at one or multiple joints of the body).

Salicylates: Medications derived from salicylic acid, including aspirin (acetylsalicylic acid).

Saturated fats: A type of dietary fat considered harmful to humans. These types of fats are solid at room temperature. They are found in all animal foods and only a few plant foods. Too much is thought to raise the level of cholesterol in the bloodstream.

Select serotonin reuptake inhibitor (SSRI): A type of drug that is used to treat depression. SSRIs slow the process by which serotonin (a substance that nerves use to send messages to one another) is reused by nerve cells that make it. This increases the amount of serotonin available for stimulating other nerves.

Serotonin: A neurotransmitter within the central nervous system.

Serotonin syndrome: A hyperserotonergic state that is a very dangerous and potentially fatal side effect of serotonergic enhancing drugs; it can have multiple psychiatric and non-psychiatric symptoms.

Sleep apnea: Cessation of breathing that occurs during sleep. Usually due to obstruction of the airway, it can also be due to inability of the brain to initiate respiration.

Sleep deprivation: A shortage of quality, undisturbed sleep that results in detrimental effects on physical and mental well-being.

Soft tissue: The ligaments, tendons, and muscles in the musculoskeletal system.

Somatic: Pertaining to the body.

SSNRIs: Serotonin and norepinephrine reuptake inhibitors (SNRIs) are a type of antidepressant medication that increases the levels of both serotonin and norepinephrine by inhibiting their reabsorption into cells in the brain.

Stimulants: Drugs that increase the activity of the sympathetic nervous system and produce a sense of euphoria or awakeness.

Subclinical hypothyroidism: A condition in which a patient has no clinical manifestation of hypothyroidism, a normal free T4 level but a mildly increased TSH level.

Substance P: A protein substance that stimulates nerve endings at an injury site and within the spinal cord, increasing pain messages.

Supination: Walking too much on the outside of your foot.

Supplements: The addition of vitamins and minerals, in a pill form, to a person's diet.

Sympathetic nervous system: The part of the autonomic nervous system that raises blood pressure and heart rate in response to stress.

Syndrome: A group of symptoms as reported by the patient and signs as detected in an examination that together are characteristic of a specific condition.

Thyroxine T4: The major hormone produced by the thyroid glands, responsible for controlling the rate of metabolism in the body, used as a measure of the thyroid glands secretory activity.

Triiodothyronine T3: Thyroid hormone similar to thyroxine but with one less iodine atom per molecule and produced in smaller quantity, is primarily produced by the peripheral conversion of T4 to T3. T3 is readily available to tissue exchange and interactions with its nuclear receptors.

Temporomandibular disorders: Conditions characterized by facial pain and restricted ability to open/move the jaw.

Temporomandibular joint (TMJ): The connecting hinge mechanism between the base of the skull (temporal bone) and the lower jaw (mandible).

Tendon: A tough cord or band of dense white fibrous connective tissue that unites a muscle with some other part (as a bone) and transmits the force that the muscle exerts.

Thoracic region: Pertaining to the chest.

Thyroid: A gland located beneath the voice box (larynx) that produces thyroid hormone. The thyroid helps regulate growth and metabolism.

tid: Medication taken three times a day.

Torque: A turning or twisting force on the body.

Toxins: Poisonous chemicals that react with specific cellular components to kill cells or to alter growth or development in undesirable ways; often harmful, even in dilute concentrations.

Tramadol: A centrally acting analgesic for the treatment of pain in fibromyalgia. Also know as Ultram.

Trans fats: Fats that are artificially created through a chemical process of the hydrogenation of oils. This solidifies the oil and limits the body's ability to regulate cholesterol. These fats are considered to be the most harmful to one's health.

Tricyclic antidepressants: A group of drugs used to relieve symptoms of depression. These drugs may also help relieve pain.

Trigeminal nerve: The main sensory nerve of the head and face, and the motor nerve of the muscles used in chewing. Also called the fifth cranial nerve.

Trigger points: 1-Places on the body where muscles and adjacent fibrous tissue (fascia) are sensitive to the touch. These areas are generally in the upper and lower back muscles, but they may occur elsewhere. 2-An area of low neurological activity that when stimulated or stressed transforms into an area of high neurological activity with referred sensations to other parts of the body.

TSH (thyroid stimulating hormone): Released by the pituitary gland to increase thyroid hormone production.

Ultracet: Ultram (tramadol) in combination with acetaminophen.

Ultrasound: An electrical modality that transmits a sound wave through an applicator into the skin to the soft tissue in order to heat the local area; for relaxing the injured tissue and/or dispersing edema.

Visceral: The internal organs of the body, specifically those within the chest (such as the heart or lungs) or abdomen (such as the liver, pancreas, or intestines).

Yoga: A system of exercises that help your control of the body and mind. It also improves your breathing and focuses the alignment of your body.

Index

A

Accommodative spasm, 147–148
Acetaminophen (Tylenol)
    explanation of, 56–57
    narcotic medications with, 63
    for temporomandibular dys-
        function pain, 114
ACTH stimulation test, 97, 99
Acupuncture
    benefits of, 14, 137–139
    for chronic pain, 133–134
    explanation of, 131–132
    for fibromyalgia, 135–136
    function of, 134–135
    modern theories of, 132–133
    procedure for, 136–137
Adderall XR, 175
Addiction, 63
ADHD/fibromyalgia and related
        symptoms, complex (AFRSC)
    case study of, 173–175
    diagnosis of, 176
    explanation of, 168, 171–172
    research needs for, 176
    treatment of, 172–173
Adjuvant therapies
    anticonvulsants as, 69–70
    antidepressants as, 64–69
    explanation of, 64

Adrenal cortex, 95
Adrenal gland, 94–95
Adrenal insufficiency (AI)
    causes of, 95
    diagnosis of, 96–97
    in fibromyalgia patients,
        98–99
    treatment of, 97–98
Adrenocorticotropin hormone
    (ACTH), 95–99
Adult ADHD Self-Report Scale
    (Adult ASRS), 170
Advanced sleep phase syndrome,
    31–32
Aerobic exercise, 191–192
Affective spectrum disorder, 172
AFRSC. See ADHD/fibromyalgia
    and related symptoms com-
    plex (AFRSC)
Aldosterone, 95
Alexander technique, 212
Allergan, 145
Allodynia, 2, 136, 155
Alosetron, 125–126
Alprazolam (Xanax), 68, 151
Alternative Treatments for
    Fibromyalgia and Chronic
    Fatigue Syndrome (Skelly
    & Helm), 243

American Academy of Pain Medicine, 62
American College of Rheumatology (ACR), 1, 42, 274
American Dental Association, 105
American Medical Association, 274
American Pain Society, 4, 62
Amiodarone, 85
Amitriptyline (Elavil)
    explanation of, 65–67
    personal experience with, 20
    side effects of, 151
Amygdala, 155
Analgesics
    eye problems as side effects of, 150
    narcotic, 62–64
    non-narcotic, 56–61
Anger
    as pain response, 155
    as stage in mourning, 158–159
Antianxiety drugs, 151
Anticonvulsants
    explanation of, 69–70
    eye problems as side effects of, 151
Antidepressants
    eye problems as side effects of, 151
    function of, 64–65, 172
    for irritable bowel syndrome, 126
    SSRI and SNRI, 67–69
    for temporomandibular dysfunction, 114
    tricyclic, 65–67
Anti-evaporates, 147
Apnea, 35
Apnea/hypopnea (AHI), 36–37
Armour thyroid, 92
Artificial tears, 145
Aspirin, 63

Attention deficit hyperactivity disorder (ADHD)
    connection between fibromyalgia and, 167–168, 171–176
    diagnosis of, 169–170
    explanation of, 168–169
    impact on health and relationships, 170–171
    myths about, 171
    statistics regarding, 168
    variations of, 170
Audio-visual entrainment (AVE), 284
Autonomic nervous system (ANS)
    divisions of, 154
    function of, 42, 153–154, 276, 280
    irritable bowel syndrome and, 121
    pain and, 156
Axial skeletal pain, 42

B

Bandage contact lenses (BCL), 146
Bargaining with God, as stage in mourning, 159
B-complex, 245
Behavioral pain management, techniques for, 160–163
Benzodiazepines, 151
Bicycle riding, 192
Binocular dysfunction (BD), 149–150
Biofeedback
    explanation of, 162
    muscle, 278–280
    to reduce muscle contractions, 115
Biofeedback Certification, 286
Body mechanics, 207, 209

Bradykinin, 8
Brain
   abnormal patterns in, 276
   pain signals and, 186
Breathing disorders, sleep-related,
      34–38
Breathing practices
   diaphragmatic, 282–283
   function of, 225–226
   yoga, 226–228
Bruxism, 12
Buckelew, S. P., 282–283

C

Calcium, 245
Calcium carbonate, 247
Calcium citrate, 247
Calcium lactate, 247
Calcium supplements, 246–247
Carbamazepine (Tegretol),
      68, 151
Carbohydrates, 240–241
Carisoprodol (Soma), 151
Centers for Disease Control, 168
Central apnea, 35
Central hypothyroidism, 84
Central nervous system
   explanation of, 153
   fibromyalgia and, 154, 193
   hypersensitivity of, 186
   pain and, 156
Central sensitization
   function of, 9
   yoga and, 224
Chang, L., 125
Cholesterol, 241
Chronic fatigue syndrome (CFS)
   accommodative spasm and,
      147–148
   dry eye disease and, 143,
      145–147

statistics regarding, 168
steroid therapy and, 98–99
vision problems in patients
   with, 141, 142
Chronic pain. See also Pain
   acupuncture for, 133–134
   behavioral techniques for,
      160–163
   emotional work to approach,
      157–160
   explanation of, 1
   foot, 264
   phenomena in patients with, 2
   sleep disorders in patients with,
      31, 38
Chronobiological disorder, 275
Ciliary muscle, 147
Circadian rhythm
   disorders in, 31–32
   explanation of, 29
Clonazepam (Klonopin), 151
Clozapine (Clozaril), 68
Coenzyme Q-10, 246
Cognitive-behavioral therapy
   (CBT), 32
Cold treatment, 189
Complex carbohydrates, 240
Computer ergonomics,
      209–211
Continuous positive airway pres-
   sure (CPAP), 37, 38
Copenhagen Declaration, 274
Corticosteroids, 151
Corticotropin, 95
Corticotropin-releasing hormone
   (CRH), 95
Cortisol, 95, 96
Costochondritis, 228
COX-1, 60
COX-2, 60
COX-2 selective NSAIDs, 60
Cryolesioning, 49

Cyclobenzaprine (Flexeril)
   explanation of, 65
   eye problems as side effect of, 151
   for temporomandibular dys-
      function, 114
Cyclooxygenase (COX), 60
Cycloplegia, 151
Cyclosporine, 145
Cytomel, 93

D

Dairy products, 244
Deep relaxation techniques, 162
Degenerative joint disease, 110
Delayed sleep phase syndrome, 31
Delegating, 217–218
Denial, 158
Dentists, 12
Depression
   case study of, 173–175
   dealing with, 14
   temporomandibular dysfunction
      and, 111
Desryll, 21
Dexamethaxone (Decadron), 151
Diagnosis
   guidelines for, 3–4
   problems related to, 20
Diagnostic tests, 7–8
Diaphragmatic breathing, 282–283
Diet. See also Nutrition
   40/30/30, 238, 242
   elements of typical, 237–238
   food sensitivities and, 243–244
   foods for healthy, 242
   foods for unhealthy, 242–243
   hypoglycemia and, 236–237
   irritable bowel syndrome and,
      125
   unhealthy, 157
40/30/30 diet, 238, 242

Dietary fats, 241–242
Dietary supplements
   calcium, 246–247
   guidelines for, 244–246
Discography, 50
Disease, nutrition and, 234–236
Donaldson, Stuart, 275, 278
Doxepin, 66
Doxycycline, 146
Drug therapy. See also specific drugs
   anticonvulsant, 69–70, 151
   antidepressant, 64–69, 114,
      126, 151, 172
   carbohydrate cravings as side
      effect of, 240
   for dry eye disease, 145–147
   eye problems as side effects of,
      150–152
   guidelines for, 4
   for insomnia, 32–34
   interactions between herbal
      products and, 61, 70
   for irritable bowel syndrome,
      125–127
   narcotic analgesic, 62–64
   non-narcotic analgesic, 56–59
   nonsteroidal anti-inflammatory,
      59–61, 114, 145–146, 150
   overview of, 55, 56, 156–157
   for temporomandibular dys-
      function, 113–114
Dry eye disease (DED)
   explanation of, 143, 144
   treatment for, 143, 145–147
Duloxetine (Cymbalta), 67,
   172, 174
Dyssomnia, 30

E

Ear discomfort, 110
Edison, Thomas, 233

Ego function regression, 163
Ego functions, 163
Electroencephalogram (EEG), 28
Electromagnetic system, 135
Elimination diet, 244
Endocrine dysfunction
    adrenal disease and, 94–99
    conclusions regarding, 99–100
    thyroid disease and, 83–94
Endocrinologists, 11
Endurance exercises, 231–232
Epidural steroid injection, 48–49
Epilepsy, 2
Ergonomics
    computer, 209–211
    explanation of, 209
Escitalopram (Lexapro), 174
Essential fatty acids, 241, 246
Exercises. See also Yoga
    aerobic, 191–192
    endurance, 231–232
    posture, 207, 208
    strengthening, 190
    stretching, 190
Eye. See also Vision problems
    exercises for, 148, 150
    function of, 142
    illustration of, 144

F

Fascia, 193, 194
Fatigue
    case study of, 173–175
    causes of, 243
Fats, dietary, 241–242
Feldenkrais, 212
Females, fight-or-flight response in, 154–155
Fibromyalgia
    autonomic dysfunction in, 276–277

brain-nervous system patterns in, 276
causes of pain in, 8–9
chronobiological disturbance in, 275
diagnosis of, 3–4
early recognition of, 273–274
examination for, 4–8
explanation of, 1–2, 41, 135–136
genetic determiners for, 14
health care system and, 166–167
information sources for, 297–303
mild, 3
mind-body therapy approaches to, 278–286
moderate, 3–4
muscle dysfunction in, 275–276
nervous system and, 153–156
onset of, 277–278
patients' perspectives on, 17–23, 73–81, 179–184
post-traumatic, 277–278
primary, 277
secondary, 277
severe, 4
statistics regarding, 3, 168
stress and, 124
symptoms of, 41–43, 53, 166, 274
treatment team for, 9–14
Fibromyalgia patients
    health history of, 188
    perpetuating factors for, 236
    pregnancy in, 251–254, 257–262
    varying perspectives of, 17–23, 73–81, 179–184, 249–262, 289–295
Fibromyalgia treatment. See also Drug therapy; Mind-body therapies; specific treatments
    advanced interventional therapies for, 51–53

cryolesioning and radiofrequency lesioning for, 49–50
development of plan for,
187–188
hazards of over-, 213–214
intervertebral disc procedures
for, 50–51
nerve blocks for, 44–47
spinal injections for, 47–49
trigger point injections for, 43–44
Fight-or-flight response, 154–155
Florinef, 98
Fluoxetine HCI (Prozac), 66,
67, 151
Folic acid, 245
Food and Drug Administration
(FDA), 90, 246
Foods. See also Diet; Nutrition
junk, 242–243
sensitivities to, 243–244
Foot problems
alignment as, 264–265
metatarsalgia as, 267
orthotics as, 268–270
overview of, 263–264
pronation and supination as,
265–266
shoes and, 270–271
weight distribution as, 267
Free thyroxine (free T4), 87, 89, 91
French Energetic School, 132–134
Functional capacity evaluation
(FCE), 8
Functional MRI (FMRI) testing, 9

G

Gabapentin (Neurontin), 69, 151
Gait abnormalities, 265–266
Gastrointestinal disorders, 60
Genetic determiners, 14

Ghrelin, 27
Glucosamine sulphate, 246
Gluten, 244
Gluten Antibody Test, 244
Glycemic index (GI), 240
Gralnek, I. M., 123
Graves' disease, 85
Grief, 157–160

H

Habituation, 2
Harvard Work Hours, Health, and
Safety Group, 27
Hashimoto's thyroiditis, 85
HDL cholesterol, 241
Headaches
in fibromyalgia patients, 45–46
temporomandibular dysfunction
and, 110–111
Health care costs, 122
Heart rate variability (HRV),
280, 281
Heart rhythm training, 280–282
Heat treatment, 189
Helm, Andrea, 243
Herbal products
drug interactions with, 61,
64, 70
for dry eye disease, 146
Histamine, 8
Hormones, 29
Hudson, James I., 172
Hydrocortisone, 97–99
Hyperpathia, 136
Hypertension, 35
Hyperthyroidism, subclinical, 94
Hypnosis, 283–284
Hypnotics, 34
Hypoadrenalism. See Adrenal
insufficiency (AI)

Hypoglycemia, 236–237
Hypothalamus, 84
Hypothyroidism
  central, 84
  common causes of, 85
  diagnosis of, 86–88
  explanation of, 84
  in fibromyalgia patients, 91–93
  subclinical, 88–89
  treatment for, 89–91

I

Ibuprofen
  for osteoarthritis in knee, 56
  for pain from temporo-
    mandibular dysfunction, 109
Information sources
  DVDs, 303
  magazines, 302
  medical journals, 302
  web sites, 297–302
Insomnia
  causes of, 30–31
  circadian rhythm, 31–32
  evaluation and management of,
    29, 32–34
  explanation of, 30
  psycho-physiologic, 31
  risk factors for, 30
International Classification of Sleep
  Disorders (ICSD), 30
Intervertebral disc precedures,
  50–51
Intradiscal electrothermal annuloplasty (IDET), 50–51
Intrathecal pump therapy, 52–53
Iodine, 85
Iron, 245
Irritable bowel syndrome (IBS)
  causes of, 120–121

demographics for, 120
diagnosis of, 243
explanation of, 119–120
in fibromyalgia patients,
  123–125
impact of, 122–123
treatment of, 125–127
Iyengar yoga, 212

J

Jacobson, Edmund, 279
Jaw, rest for, 114–115
Joint capsules, 194
Joint mobilization, 193
Journaling, 215–216
Journal of Musculoskeletal Pain, 302

K

Kafka, Franz, 166
Kappa opioid receptor, 62

L

Laboratory tests
  for adrenal insufficiency, 96–97
  function of, 5
  for thyroid hormone levels,
    86–88
LDL cholesterol, 241
Leptin, 27
Levothyroxine (synthetic T4), 90, 92
Ligaments, 194
Liotrex (Thyrolar), 92
Lithium, 85
Living With Fibromyalgia DVD, 303
Lorazepam (Ativan), 151
Low back pain, 47–48
Low blood sugar, 236–237

M

Magazines, for fibromyalgia information, 302
Magnesium, 245, 246
Malic acid, 245
Massage therapists, 11, 195
Maximum heart rate (MHR), 191–192
Medical history forms, 5
Medication contracts, 64
Melatonin, 29
Memory, 162–163
The Metamorphosis (Kafka), 165–166
Metatarsalgia, 267
Methocarbamol (Robaxin), 151
Mild fibromyalgia, 3, 9
Milnacipran (Ixel), 67
Mind-body therapies
    advantages of, 284–286
    audio-visual entrainment as, 284
    diaphragmatic breathing as, 282–283
    explanation of, 273
    heart rhythm training as, 280–282
    hypnosis and self-hypnosis as, 283–284
    muscle biofeedback as, 278–280
    neurofeedback as, 284
Minerals
    for dry eye disease, 146
    function of, 242
    for muscle function, 245
Mobilization
    joint, 193
    soft tissue, 193–194
Modafinil (Provigil), 174
Moderate fibromyalgia
    central sensitization in, 9
    explanation of, 3–4

Moist heat, 115
Morphine, 21
Mourning process, 13, 157–160
Mucomimetics, 147
Multidisciplinary treatment, 10
Mu opioid receptor, 62
Muscle biofeedback, 278–280
Muscle fibers, 193
Muscle relaxants, 114, 151
Muscles
    abnormal patterns in, 275–276
    causes of pain in, 8–9
    evaluating texture and feel of, 188
    intestine, 121
    relaxation of, 11
    strengthening exercises for, 190
    structural abnormalities in, 186
    temporomandibular dysfunction and, 109
    trigger points in, 8, 194
Muscle spasms, 115
Musculoskeletal disorders, 104–118
Mydriasis, 151
Myofascial pain dysfunction syndrome, 44, 112

N

Narcotic analgesics
    adverse effects of, 62–63
    availability of, 63–64
    drug interactions with, 64
    explanation of, 62
    medication contracts for, 64
    precautions regarding, 64
Nasal continuous positive airway pressure (CPAP), 37, 38
National Fibromyalgia Association, 220
Naturethyroid, 92

Nerve blocks, 44–47
Nerve cell stimulation, 132
Nervous system
　abnormal patterns in, 276
　autonomic, 42, 121, 153–154,
　　156, 276, 280
　central, 153, 154, 156, 186, 193
　parasympathetic, 154
　sympathetic, 133, 154–155,
　　276–277, 280
Neurofeedback, 284
Neuromodulation, 51–53
Neurotransmitters, 132, 133
Neurovasoactive substances, 8
Night guards, 113
Non-narcotic analgesics
　acetaminophen, 56–57
　nonsteroidal anti-inflammatory,
　　59–61
　tramadol, 57–59
Non-rapid eye movement sleep
　(NREM) sleep, 28–29
Nonsteroidal anti-inflammatory
　drugs (NSAIDs)
　adverse effects of, 60–61
　drug interactions with, 61
　explanation of, 59–60
　eye problems as side effects
　　of, 150
　ocular, 145–146
　precautions regarding, 61
　for temporomandibular dys-
　　function, 114
Norepindphrine, 67, 172
Nutrients
　carbohydrates as, 240–241
　fats as, 241–242
　protein as, 238–239
　vitamins and minerals as, 242
Nutrition. See also Diet
　disease and, 234–236

hypoglycemia and, 236–237
importance of, 233–234
Nutritionals, for dry eye disease,
　146–147
Nutritionists, 13

O

Obstructive sleep apnea
　(OSA)/hypopnea syndrome
　diagnosis of, 36–37
　explanation of, 35–36
　treatment of, 37
Occipital nerve block, 46
Occipital neuralgia, 45, 46
Ocular nonsteroidal anti-inflam-
　matory drugs (NSAIDs),
　145–146
Office of Nutritional Products,
　Labeling, and Dietary Sup-
　plements (ONPLDS), 246
Off-the-shelf orthotics, 269–270
Omega 3 fatty acids, 146–147, 241
Omega 6 fatty acids, 241
Opiates, 62, 133
Opioid receptors, 62
Opioids, 62
Oral orthotics, 113
Orthotics
　explanation of, 113, 268–269
　off-the-shelf, 269–270
Orthotists, 12, 263
Ostalecki, Sharon, 256
Osteoporosis, 246

P

Pain. See also Chronic pain
　axial skeletal, 42
　facial, 103–117
　in fibromyalgia, 8–9, 42–43

low back, 47–48
muscle, 109
patient perspective on, 17–23
sympathetic nervous system
and, 155
wide-spread, 1
Pain management
behavioral techniques for,
160–163
challenges to, 187
drug therapy for, 4, 56–70,
113–114, 156–157
emotional work for, 157–160
physical therapy treatments for,
189–194
Pain psychologists. *See* Rehabilita-
tion/pain psychologists
Parafon Forte DSC (Chlorzoxazone), 114
Parasympathetic nervous
system, 154
Patching, eye, 149–150
Patient education
in body mechanics, 207–209
in ergonomics, 209–211
need for, 195–196
by physical therapists, 201
in proper posture, 202–207
self-management through, 215
Patient history, 188
Paxil, 66
Percutaneous disc decompression,
50–51
Phenelzine (Nardil), 66
Phenytoin (Dilantin), 68
Physiatrists, 3, 4
Physical dependence, 63
Physical examination
by physical therapists, 187–188
procedure for initial, 5–6
Physical therapists
education role of, 195–196

objective findings by, 189
physical examination by,
187–188
posture evaluation by, 206–207
selection criteria for, 195
Physical therapy
function of, 11, 185, 212
phases of, 196–199
physical examination by,
196–199
for temporomandibular dysfunction, 115
treatment plans for, 189–194
Pituitary gland, 84
Polysomnographers, 12
Polysomnography (PSY), 36
Positive airway pressure (PAP), 37
Post-traumatic fibromyalgia,
277–278
Posture
difficulties related to, 205, 209
evaluation of, 206–207
exercises for, 207, 208
guidelines for, 202, 207
illustrations of, 203, 204
Potassium, 245
Pramipexole (Mirapex), 172–173
Prednisone, 151
Pregabalin (Lyrica), 69
Pregnancy, 251–254, 257–262
Presbyopia, 147
Primary fibromyalgia, 277
Prioritizing, 218–219
Prisms, 149
Progressive muscle relaxation
(PMR), 279–280
Pronation, 265
Prostaglandins, 8
Protein, 238–239
Psychiatrists, 14
Psychologists. *See* Rehabilitation/
pain psychologists

Psycho-physiologic insomnia, 31
Psychostimulants, 172
Punctal plugs, 146

R

Radiofrequency lesioning, 50
Rapid eye movement (REM) sleep, 28, 29
Raynaud's disease, 155
Rechtschaffen and Kales scoring system (R&K system), 28
Recommended Dietary Allowance (RDA), 239, 244
Referred sensory phenomena (RSP), 112
Rehabilitation/pain psychologists, 13, 21
Relaxation response, 281–282
Relaxation techniques, 162
Restasis, 145

S

Sadness
    function of, 13
    as stage in mourning, 159–160
Secondary fibromyalgia, 277
Secretagogues, 147
Selective serotonin reuptake inhibitors (SSRIs)
    drug interactions with, 68–69
    explanation of, 67–68
    side effects of, 240
Selegiline (Eldepryl), 66
Selenium, for dry eye disease, 146
Self-hypnosis, 283–284
Self-management
    delegating as, 217–218
    fibromyalgia knowledge and, 215
    function of, 213–214, 220–221

journaling as, 215–216
    prioritizing as, 218–219
    saying "no" as element of, 216–217
    stress reduction as, 219–220
    support groups for, 220
Serotonergic inhibitory brainstem pathways, 2
Serotonin
    absorption of, 67
    irritable bowel syndrome and, 121
    morphine and, 21
    use of, 172
Serotonin norepinephrine reuptake inhibitors (SNRIs), 67–68, 155
Serotonin syndrome, 58
Sertraline (Zoloft), 21, 22, 66, 67, 151, 174
Severe fibromyalgia, 4, 9
Shoes, 270–271
Shoulder blade stretch exercise, 208
Skelly, Mari, 243
Sleep
    circadian rhythms and, 29
    function of, 25–26
    hormonal changes during, 29
    stages and architecture of, 27–29
Sleep apnea, 12, 34
Sleep apnea (OSA) syndrome, 34
Sleep disorders
    brain and nervous system patterns and, 276
    breathing-related, 34–38
    categories of, 30
    effects of, 26–27
    insomnia as, 30–34
    melatonin and, 29
    in patients with chronic pain, 31, 38

Sleep-related breathing disorders
    explanation of, 34
    obstructive sleep apnea syn-
        drome as, 35–37
    snoring as, 34–35
    treatment of, 37–38
Sleep studies, 12
Slouching, 206
Slow-transport system, 2
Soft tissue mobilization, 193–194
Spinal cord stimulation, 52
Spinal injections, 47–49
Stella, G., 279
Stellate ganglion, 46–47
Stellate ganglion block, 47
Steroid eye drops, 145–146
Strengthening exercises, 190
Stress
    fibromyalgia and, 124
    guidelines to reduce, 219–220
    irritable bowel syndrome
        and, 124
    temporomandibular dysfunction
        and, 115
Stretching exercises, 190
Subclinical hyperthyroidism,
    88–89, 94
Sugar, 244
Supination, 265
Support groups, 220
Suprachiasmatic nucleus
    (SCN), 29
Surface electromyogram (sEMG)
    biofeedback training, 11
Sympathetic nervous system, 133,
    154–155, 276–277, 280

T

Tai chi chuan, 212
Teeth clenching, 111
Tegaserod, 125–126

Temporomandibular dysfunction
    (TMD)
    chewing muscles associated
        with, 107–108
    degenerative joint disease associ-
        ated with, 110
    explanation of, 12, 104–105, 255
    internal derangement of TMJ
        and, 109–110
    muscle pain and, 109
    neck muscles associated with, 108
    self-management of, 116
    specialists for, 117
    symptoms of, 103–104,
        108–112
    treatment of, 112–116
Temporomandibular joint (TMJ)
    anatomy of, 105–106
    ear symptoms and, 110
    facial pain and, 111
    headache and, 110–111
    muscles associated with,
        107–108
Tetracyclines, 146
Thalamus, 155
Theophylline, 68
Thoracic outlet syndrome, 19, 20
Thoracic stretch exercise, 208
Three-part breath, 227–228
Thyroid disease
    abnormal thyroid physiology
        and, 84–85
    hyperthyroidism, 94
    hypothyroidism, 86–91
    hypothyroidism in fibromyalgia
        patients, 91–94
Thyroidectomy, 85
Thyroid gland, 94–95
Thyroid-hormone resistance syn-
    dromes, 85
Thyroid stimulating hormone
    (TSH), 29, 87–91

Thyrotropin, 84
Thyrotropin-releasing hormone (TRH), 84
Thyroxine (T4), 83–84, 87, 90, 92–94
Time management, 218–219
TMJ. *See* Temporomandibular dysfunction (TMD); Temporomandibular joint (TMJ)
TMJ appliances, 113
Tolerance, 63
Tooth grinding, 12
Training index (TI), 192
Tramadol
    acetaminophen with, 57
    explanation of, 58–59
Transdisciplinary treatment, 10
Tranylcypromine (Parnate), 66
Travell, Janet, 44
Treatment team
    function of, 9
    members of, 11–14
    multidisciplinary and transdisciplinary, 10
TRH test, 88
Tricyclic antidepressants
    adverse effects of, 65
    dosing for, 65–66
    drug interactions with, 66–67
    explanation of, 65
    for irritable bowel syndrome, 126
    precautions for, 66
    side effects of, 240
Trigger point injections
    explanation of, 43–44
    illustration of, 45
Trigger points
    acupuncture and, 137, 138
    explanation of, 8, 194
    location of, 6, 7

myofascial pain dysfunction syndrome and, 44
Triiodothyronine (T3), 83–85, 87, 88, 92–94

U

Ultram, 21, 22
Ultrasound therapy, 190
Upper airway resistance syndrome, 35

V

Vascular headaches, 45
Venlafaxine (Effexor), 67–68, 172
Vicodin, 21
Vision problems
    accommodative spasm, 147–148
    binocular dysfunction, 149–150
    dry eye disease, 143–147
    in fibromyalgia patients, 14
    as medication side effects, 150–152
    overview of, 142–143
Visualization, benefits of, 230
Vitamin B_1, 245
Vitamin B_6, 245
Vitamin B_{12}, 245
Vitamin D, 247
Vitamins
    for dry eye disease, 146
    for fibromyalgia patients, 245
    function of, 242

W

Web sites, for fibromyalgia information, 297–302
Weight distribution, 267
Wellness, 235–236

Wessely, S., 124
Westhroid, 92
Wide-spread pain, 1
Withdrawal reflex, 155
World Health Organization
(WHO), 56, 274

Y

Yoga
benefits of, 14, 212, 224–225
breathing practices for, 225–228
for endurance, 231–232
explanation of, 223
for flare-ups, 230–231
for individuals in remission, 232
Yoga classes, 230
Yoga for Healing (DVD), 231
Yoga postures
explanation of, 228–229
guidelines for practicing,
229–230

Z

Zinc, 146